Hypothyroidism

Rudolf Hoermann • Johannes W. Dietrich
Editors

Hypothyroidism

A Paradigm Shift

Springer

Editors
Rudolf Hoermann
Department of General Internal Medicine, Gastroenterology and Endocrinology
[Retired] Klinikum Lüdenscheid
Lüdenscheid, Germany

Johannes W. Dietrich
Diabetes, Endocrinology and Metabolism Section, Department of Medicine
St. Josef-Hospital, Ruhr University Hospitals
Bochum, Germany

ISBN 978-981-96-3681-5 ISBN 978-981-96-3682-2 (eBook)
https://doi.org/10.1007/978-981-96-3682-2

This Springer imprint is published by the registered company Springer Nature Singapore Pte Ltd.
The registered company address is: 152 Beach Road, #21-01/04 Gateway East, Singapore 189721, Singapore

In memoriam John Edward M. Midgley

Preface

Before the recognition of its etiology as a disease of the thyroid, hypothyroidism was first described as a clinical syndrome manifesting with a characteristic spectrum of symptoms. The diagnosis of hypothyroidism rapidly gained momentum after the appearance of biochemical thyroid function testing, becoming thereby one of the most frequently diagnosed and treated diseases in the world. This remarkable development was pushed by the convenient and sensitive measurement of pituitary thyroid stimulating hormone (thyrotropin, TSH) as an indirect marker of thyroid function. In the process, TSH achieved a pre-eminent position on its own by assuming a direct and proportional linkage to thyroid function. This culminated in defining an entirely new class of disease and treatment target, termed subclinical hypothyroidism, reliant solely on an abnormality of a single biochemical parameter. As all of this occurred in a short period of time, guidelines emerged as a valuable but over-promoted driver of unprecedented influence, which replaced individual treatment choices made between patient and doctor. The gross dissociation of this strategy from individual patient care has long been overlooked, though voices of discontent have increasingly expressed dissatisfaction with the standard current diagnosis and treatment paradigm. Recent developments and particularly advances in our understanding of hypothalamic-pituitary-thyroid regulation make it necessary to scale back on the assumed universal utility of TSH as the most reliable thyroid function test. The need to revisit and update long-held beliefs in how we diagnose and treat thyroid disease has now become an urgent task.

In this book, the diagnosis and treatment of hypothyroidism is approached from a different perspective that shifts the narrative and paradigm of the disease. We introduce the concept of relational stability between FT4, FT3, and TSH and thoroughly examine the role of thyroid hormone homeostasis including FT3 as a main determinant of thyroid health and disease. In doing so, we relied heavily on our own experience and decades of published research from our group to address the major issues of dispute in the treatment of hypothyroidism. Together with the patient presentation and conditionality of the expressed biochemistry, our approach portrays a unique view of the importance of thyroid hormone regulation beyond statistical aggregation. This allows personalized criteria in diagnostic and therapeutic decision-making. We summarize recent physiological advances together with accepted standards in a structured format and translate them into practical care. This critical reappraisal and novel perspective should be of interest to a wide audience in thyroidology and beyond as it shifts the paradigm on the diagnosis and treatment of hypothyroidism.

Yandina, Australia Rudolf Hoermann
Bochum, Germany Johannes W. Dietrich

Competing Interests

Johannes W. Dietrich is co-owner of the intellectual property rights for the patent "System and Method for Deriving Parameters for Homeostatic Feedback Control of an Individual" (Singapore Institute for Clinical Sciences, Biomedical Sciences Institutes, Application Number 201208940-5, WIPO number WO/2014/088516). Rudolf Hoermann, John E. Midgley, and Mark J. Pekker have no conflicts of interest to declare that are relevant to the content of this book or a chapter.

Acknowledgments

We would like to acknowledge the support of our colleague and coworker Rolf Larisch over many years. We also wish to thank Tania Smith, Thyroid Patients Canada and Peter Warmingham, Thyroid UK for valuable discussions.

Ethics Approval Not applicable.
No primary studies were conducted.

About This book

This book builds on advances in our understanding of the regulation of the hypothalamic-pituitary-thyroid axis and homeostasis of the thyroid system. From this perspective, it provides a new conceptual and practical framework to address current issues in the diagnosis and treatment of hypothyroidism. It calls for and explains a necessary shift in our approach to the prevalent disease. This should be of interest to a wide readership, medical professionals and interested patients alike.

Contents

List of Figures

List of Tables

Chapter 1
Hypothyroidism

Rudolf Hoermann and Johannes W. Dietrich

1.1 Definition

Hypothyroidism has been traditionally defined in older textbooks as a diminished effect and/or response of thyroid hormones on organs and tissues [1]. This is understandable, given the many steps in the pathway finally leading to the cellular actions of thyroid hormones. In turn, this influences a plethora of energetic and metabolic reactions in the human body [2, 3]. Depending on the severity of the hormone deficit the condition of hypothyroidism depicts a broad disease spectrum. The manifestation of the clinical disease comes with a multitude of more or less characteristic signs and symptoms, caused and accompanied by the development of the biochemical abnormalities [4–6].

More recent definitions restricted the classical definition to the most prevalent form of thyroid failure, termed *primary hypothyroidism* [7]. According to this classification, the spectrum of hypothyroidism extends from a latent or subclinical form

R. Hoermann (✉)
Yandina, QLD, Australia

Department of General Internal Medicine, Gastroenterology and Endocrinology, [Retired] Klinikum Lüdenscheid, Lüdenscheid, Germany
e-mail: rudolf.hoermann@gmail.com

J. W. Dietrich
Diabetes, Endocrinology and Metabolism Section, Department of Medicine, St. Josef-Hospital, Ruhr University Hospitals, Bochum, Germany

Centre for Diabetes Technology (ZDT), Catholic Hospitals Bochum, Bochum, Germany

Centre for Rare Endocrine Diseases (ZSEK), Ruhr Center for Rare Diseases (CeSER), Ruhr University of Bochum and Witten/Herdecke University, Bochum, Germany

Centre for Thyroid Medicine (ZSM), Ruhr University of Bochum, Bochum, Germany
e-mail: johannes.dietrich@ruhr-uni-bochum.de

R. Hoermann, J. W. Dietrich (eds.), *Hypothyroidism*,
https://doi.org/10.1007/978-981-96-3682-2_1

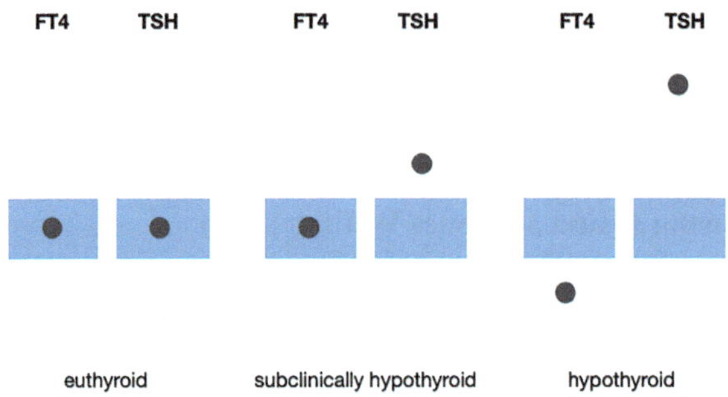

Fig. 1.1 Classification of primary hypothyroidism
In euthyroidism, both FT4 and TSH are found within their respective reference ranges, while subclinical hypothyroidism is defined by an elevated TSH with FT4 in the reference range and overt hypothyroidism by the combination of a low FT4 and high TSH concentration. Blue boxes indicate the respective reference ranges

of hypothyroidism to overt hypothyroidism. Subclinical hypothyroidism can only be recognised indirectly via impaired thyroid hormone control and elevation of the pituitary hormone, thyroid-stimulating hormone (TSH), with FT4 concentrations still being in the reference range. In overt hypothyroidism, FT4 concentrations in the blood have declined below the lower limit of the reference range, and TSH is elevated (Fig. 1.1). In rare but extreme manifestations, hypothyroidism aggravates to the life-threatening myxedematous coma.

1.2 Epidemiology

Hypothyroidism is a prevalent disease in the adult population, and its incidence increases with age. Population prevalence is estimated to be 1–3% for overt hypothyroidism and 5–10% including subclinical hypothyroidism [8–17]. The disease shows a female preponderance, being at least 4 times more frequent in women, compared to men.

1.3 Aetiology

The clinical syndrome of hypothyroidism arises in the majority of cases from an inadequate supply of the body with thyroid hormones due to a significant reduction of the synthesis and secretion of the two main thyroid hormones, T4 and T3, by the thyroid gland (Table 1.1). This shortage is mostly related to thyroid gland failure or *primary hypothyroidism* [7]. The cause of primary hypothyroidism may be distinguished from *secondary or tertiary hypothyroidism*, which is caused by a primary deficiency in the pituitary or hypothalamus, respectively [18]. The low level of basal

Table 1.1 Causes of hypothyroidism

Primary hypothyroidism
Inborn errors of developments Thyroid dysgenesis, aplasia, dysplasia Ectopic thyroid to the root of the tongue
Deficiencies in iodine metabolism affecting iodine transport, thyroid peroxidase, thyroglobulin synthesis, iodine–tyrosyl coupling, deiodinases, thyroglobulin release
Transient hypothyroidism of the newborn due to blocking-type TSH receptor antibodies (TSHR Abs) transferred from a mother with Graves' disease to the foetus Iodine deficiency (severe) Iodine excess (iodine-induced hypothyroidism) Anti-thyroid compounds
Autoimmune thyroiditis With thyroid atrophy (Ord's disease) With thyroid hypertrophy (original Hashimoto's thyroiditis)
Other forms of thyroiditis Subacute de Quervain's thyroiditis Post-partum thyroiditis Silent thyroiditis Riedel's thyroiditis Cytokine-induced thyroiditis COVID-19-associated subacute thyroiditis
Hypothyroidism due to therapeutic interventions and environmental toxins Thyroidectomy Radioiodine treatment including late manifestation 10 years after the treatment Radiation to the neck area Use of anti-thyroid drugs, lithium, amiodarone, interferon and checkpoint inhibitors Exposure to endocrine-disrupting chemicals
Rare diseases of the thyroid Amyloidosis, sarcoidosis, lymphoma and other thyroid tumours
Secondary hypothyroidism
Pituitary deficiency, pituitary tumours, hypophysitis
Tertiary hypothyroidism
Deficiency or diseases of the hypothalamus
Thyroid hormone transport deficiency
MCT8 deficiency (Allan-Herndon-Dudley syndrome)
Reduced sensitivity to thyroid hormone
Thyroid hormone resistance syndromes, TSH-receptor resistance, G-protein abnormalities (Albright dystrophy)

secretion of the thyroid gland is insufficient for the maintenance of thyroid hormone homeostasis and proper functioning of the organism at a healthy level [19]. The thyroid gland therefore requires further activation by hypothalamic TRH and, subsequently, pituitary TSH to appropriately raise the levels of the hormones to the euthyroid range to achieve a clinical state that meets the normal needs of the organism.

A lack of responsiveness of the target organs to sufficient amounts of circulating thyroid hormones can be a less frequent cause of hypothyroidism, due to some—not all—*syndromes of reduced sensitivity to thyroid hormone*, formerly known as acquired or inherited thyroid hormone resistance syndrome [20].

1.4 Primary Hypothyroidism

Primary hypothyroidism is the most prevalent functional thyroid disease in the population. Its aetiology is primarily a chronic underlying autoimmune process, resulting in an ongoing inflammatory reaction with slowly progressive destruction of thyroid tissue [5]. The name of this clinical disease is autoimmune thyroiditis, *Hashimoto's thyroiditis* (if the thyroid gland is enlarged) or *Ord's disease* (if the thyroid gland is atrophic). The sequelae of how the disease may evolve varies considerably, from (a) the presence of the autoimmune process in the absence of any functional consequences to (b) a functionally compensated state with slightly elevated TSH levels and (c) eventually the transition into biochemically recognisable hypothyroidism and (d) the development of apparent clinical symptoms. As in any chronic disease, patients may transit through the different phases more gradually, though sometimes the onset occurs more rapidly. However, in some cases, it is possible that the process may stop or even reverse at early stage. The immunological disease frequently leaves its typical hallmark on the thyroid gland, which can be seen as a hypoechogenic pattern in ultrasound. Glands are mostly subject to shrinkage (atrophy), but gland hypertrophy is also possible, as featured in the original description of this disease by Hakaru Hashimoto [21]. Autoimmune markers such as thyroid peroxidase (TPO) antibodies are prevalent, both before and after the onset of hypothyroidism as a functional disease [22]. They may however decline or be absent in patients with long-standing chronic disease.

Apart from the prevalent immunological disorder, acute and subacute infections with various pathogens may result in other forms of thyroiditis. Those display a more abrupt onset and distinct clinical pattern, such as the painful subacute de Quervain's thyroiditis with elevated infection markers (Table 1.1). A more recent manifestation is the COVID-19-associated subacute thyroiditis [23].

The second most frequent cause of hypothyroidism is the result of therapeutic interventions, such as thyroidectomy, radioiodine treatment, radiation of the neck, treatment with immune checkpoint inhibitors, medication with certain drugs that interfere with thyroid function [5, 15], severe iodine deficiency or iodine excess and endocrine-disrupting chemicals [24].

1.4.1 Pathogenesis of Thyroid Autoimmune Disease

Autoimmune thyroiditis, also known as Hashimoto's thyroiditis, and *Graves' disease* are the two most common immunological disorders affecting thyroid function and morphology [22, 25–28]. While Graves' disease usually causes thyroid hyperfunction, autoimmune thyroiditis leads to hypothyroidism in the long term. The immunological disorders affect 5–10% of the population with a strong female preponderance. The two diseases share multiple similarities, but they also differ in some important properties [29] (Table 1.2). Both are associated with other autoimmune diseases [30].

In Graves' disease, the immune system takes control of thyroid function. However, unlike hypothalamic-pituitary-thyroid control, the stimulation by the immune system lacks feedback regulation, allowing for the overproduction of thyroid hormones and the development of hyperthyroidism [31]. A key feature in the pathogenesis of Graves' disease is the production of autoantibodies, capable of binding to and activating the human TSH receptor, termed TSHR Ab [32] (Fig. 1.2). Stimulating TSHR Ab, also termed TSAb, mimics the actions of the pituitary hormone TSH, but in an uncontrolled fashion, leading to hyperthyroidism [33]. Hypothyroid Graves' disease is a rare subform originating from the formation of blocking TSH receptor antibodies (iTSHR Abs). Thyroid-specific auto-antigens include the TSH receptor, the key enzyme of thyroid hormone production thyroid peroxidase, targeted by thyroid peroxidase antibodies (TPO Ab), and the thyroglobulin molecule, corresponding thyroglobulin antibodies (Tg Ab) bind to. These autoantigens and antibodies are shared between Graves' disease and autoimmune thyroiditis, albeit in different frequencies, with TSHR Abs being most prevalent in Graves' disease, and TPO Ab in patients with autoimmune thyroiditis (Table 1.2).

In contrast to the actions of B cells producing the stimulatory antibodies in Graves' disease, in autoimmune thyroiditis autoreactive T cells destroy functional thyroid tissue, leading to scarring and loss of function, eventually resulting in hypothyroidism [34]. They cause a chronic inflammatory response with a typical inhomogeneous hypoechogenic pattern that is apparent in thyroid imaging by ultrasound.

Table 1.2 Similarities and dissimilarities between autoimmune thyroiditis and Graves' disease

Shared properties
Immunological origin (thyroid autoimmune disease)
Shared antigens
Concordant familial risk
Higher prevalence in women, incidence ratio of 1–4:6
Increasing incidence with age, nearly linearly, peaking at age 50 in women and 60 in men
Overlap syndromes and transitions between the two diseases
Distinct properties
Caused by different immunological mechanisms
Different immunological key targets, thyroid peroxidase and thyroglobulin in autoimmune thyroiditis vs human TSH receptor in Graves' disease
Destructive thyroid disease in autoimmune thyroiditis vs functional thyroid disease in Graves' disease
Different clinical course, slow progression of autoimmune thyroiditis vs abrupt onset of Graves' disease
Different prognosis with infrequent remissions in autoimmune thyroiditis vs frequent remissions in Graves' disease

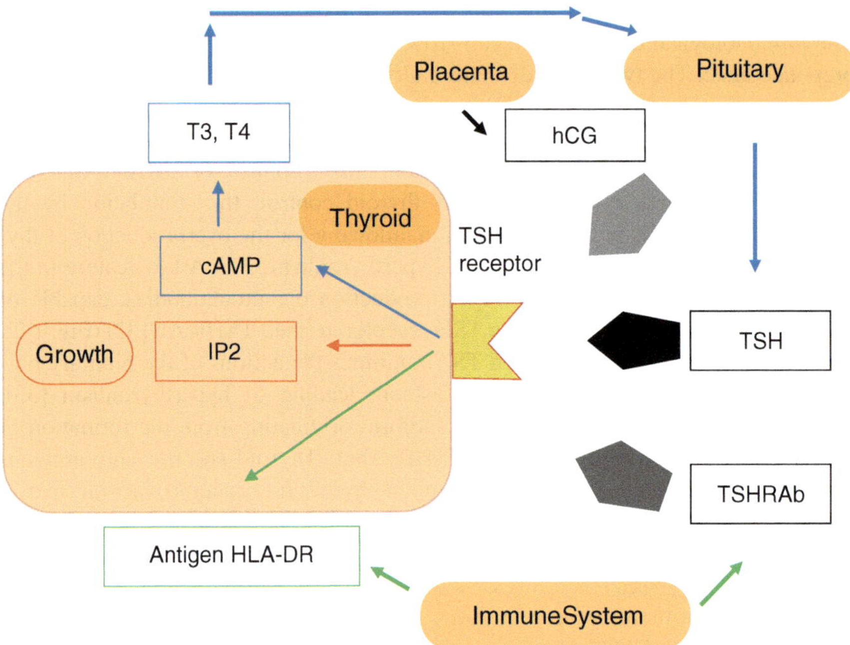

Fig. 1.2 Role of TSH receptor in thyroid function, growth and thyroid immunity
The human TSH receptor is activated by the pituitary hormone TSH, and other TSH receptor agonists such as the pregnancy hormone human chorionic gonadotropin (hCG) and TSH receptor antibodies (TSHR Abs) present in Graves' disease. Receptor activation, in turn, activates several distinct pathways to increase not only thyroid function but also thyroid growth and altered surface antigen expression

The chronic destructive immune process leads to a slowly progressive atrophy of the thyroid gland, although the process may sometimes come to a halt at any stage, or as stated earlier can even be associated with glandular hypertrophy instead of shrinkage of the gland. In some cases, a short initial phase of thyrotoxicosis (referred to as Hashitoxicosis) is observed, which usually transitions into primary hypothyroidism. The hypertrophic variant of the autoimmune disease was the one first described by Hashimoto [21]. While the name Hashimoto's disease has been originally reserved for the autoimmune disease presenting with goitre, the terms autoimmune thyroiditis and Hashimoto's thyroiditis are now mostly used synonymously.

It is important to understand the dual role of the pituitary and its hormone, TSH, on both thyroid function and thyroid growth. TSH induces thyroid follicular cells (thyrocytes) to synthesise and secrete the main thyroid hormones, T4 and T3 and to proliferate, for the gland to grow [35]. In turn, thyroid hormones exert a negative feedback on the production of TSH to maintain the homeostasis of hormone levels and gland sizes of the pituitary and thyroid [33]. Importantly, this circuit equally supports control of the size of the thyroid gland, thereby closely linking cell growth and cell function [36, 37]. Both are achieved by the same TSH signal. Yet thyroid growth responds at a slower timescale, compared to thyroid function, enlarging the thyroid, known as goitre, to increase thyroid hormone production sites and facilitate the achievement of thyroid hormone homeostasis. Apart from enhanced TSH stimulation, the formation of goitre occurs when concentrations of iodine for thyroid hormone synthesis are low [38]. This may increase the sensitivity of thyrocytes to the stimulatory actions of TSH. Reciprocally increasing and decreasing gland masses of the thyroid and pituitary produce a shifted cycle in the release of TSH and thyroid hormones, which forms the basis of a seasonal pattern that can be observed in circulating TSH and thyroid hormone concentrations in many species including, albeit to a lesser degree, in humans [39, 40]. This mechanism is at the origin of a memory effect of the past, known as hysteresis [36, 41] (Sect. 5.3.8). Understanding pituitary-thyroid linkage and the phenomenon of hysteresis becomes clinically relevant when interpreting TSH measurements in the context of thyroid function testing [42, 43].

Autoimmune surveillance *theory* suggests that regulatory T cells may have a role in healthy individuals as well [29, 34]. According to this theory, they control and eliminate mutant cells that tend to increase sensitivity to the TSH signal, thereby increasing both hormone secretion and proliferation (Fig. 1.2). Such mutant cells are frequently caused by mutations in the TSH receptor or the receptor-coupled G protein [35]. They grow into clones, clinically known as toxic thyroid nodules or hyperfunctioning adenomas. The overactive clones are immunologically recognisable, because the TSH receptor and TSH pathway are linked to the expression of immunological markers such as HLA-DR and intracellular adhesion molecule 1 in thyroid follicular cells [29, 44] (Fig. 1.2). In susceptible individuals, these T cells can trigger a broader response against specific thyroid antigens, namely the human TSH receptor, the enzyme thyroid peroxidase and the thyroglobulin molecule. A shared origin may explain similarities in incidence and risk factors between autoimmune thyroiditis and Graves' disease, despite their different functional and clinical phenotypes [29] (Table 1.2). We note that a transition between the two opposing functional entities is possible in a patient, and a repeated shift between the two entities has also been occasionally observed.

Notably, blockade of the human TSH receptor has been experimentally shown to inhibit thyroid function, thyroid growth including malignant growth and metastasis and expression of immunological surface markers [44–47].

The *pathogenesis* of the underlying autoimmune process that causes thyroid gland failure in autoimmune thyroiditis is as yet only partly understood. A main pathological feature in autoimmune thyroiditis is the tissue infiltration by lymphocytes. The lymphatic cells are autoreactive, recognising thyroid-specific antigens such as the enzyme thyroid peroxidase, the molecule thyroglobulin, the TSH receptor (more so in Graves' disease) and the sodium symporter [34, 48]. Dendritic cells, macrophages and B-lymphocytes are instrumental in presenting the antigens to maturing CD4+ and cytotoxic CD8+ lymphocytes, which, in turn, interact with neutrophils, regulatory T cells and natural killer cells [27]. The clinical manifestation towards autoimmune thyroiditis or Graves' disease depends on the balance between TH1 and TH2 helper cell subpopulations, as well as the presence of TH17 cells (which secrete the cytokine IL-17), antigen-presenting cells and the cytokine profile that dominates in the thyroid tissue [49]. The pathological T-cell response arises on a genetic basis (HLA-DR3 and HLA DR5) in conjunction with endogenous (regulatory T-cell deficiency, oestrogens, polycystic ovary syndrome) and exogenous risk factors (viral infection, stressors including psychological stress, high dose of iodine, cytokines) and other modulators (e.g. nicotine [50]). The subsequent cytotoxic immune reaction increases the production of specific cytokines such as interferon-gamma, interleukin-1 and tumour necrosis factor, leading to a predominant antibody-dependent cell-mediated cytotoxicity observed in autoimmune thyroiditis. Thyrocytes become intimately involved in the pathogenetic process when triggered by antibodies and cytokines released from lymphatic cells to both present antigens on their surface and release pro-inflammatory mediators themselves, thereby amplifying and perpetuating the autoimmune response [34] (Fig. 1.2). This process is slow, but ongoing, thereby progressively destroying functional thyroid follicles. FAS-mediated apoptosis of thyrocytes may further add to the tissue destruction. Thyroid hormones, on the other hand, influence the development of innate and adaptive immunity.

Notably, not every patient with apparent autoimmune thyroiditis progresses to thyroid gland failure, requiring substitution with thyroid hormones. The onset of the autoimmune process may pre-date the development of the clinically apparent disease and manifestation of hypothyroidism by many years, even decades, rapid progression being an exception. Because follicle destruction is a key process in autoimmune thyroiditis, an initially thyrotoxic phase may occasionally occur due to abrupt release of thyroid hormones into the circulation (Hashitoxicosis). This phenomenon can otherwise be more typically seen in patients with de Quervain's thyroiditis.

In a subgroup of patients with autoimmune thyroiditis (approx. 10%), blocking-type TSHR Abs are pathophysiologically dominant, rather than the expression of destructive cytotoxicity. Importantly, this variant of autoimmune thyroiditis may prove reversible over time, not requiring life-long hormone substitution. It has been observed more commonly in certain inflammatory conditions, e.g. hidradenitis [51].

Fluctuating Graves' disease describes a disease where the functional manifestation may shift between hypothyroidism and hyperthyroidism, either depending on the dominance of a stimulatory or inhibitory TSH receptor antibody spectrum or the temporal superposition of positive and negative feedback loops in the context of dynamical compensation [52].

Autoimmune thyroiditis may occasionally coexist with other thyroid diseases. The presence of autoimmune thyroid disease in combination with thyroid autonomy (toxic adenoma) is termed *Marine-Lenhart syndrome* [53]. The expression of hypothyroidism may be temporarily variable and self-correcting in these conditions.

References

1. Braverman LE, Utiger RD. Introduction to hypothyroidism. In: Braverman LE, Utiger RD, editors. The thyroid. J.B. Lippincott Company; 1991. p. 919–20.
2. Cheng S-Y, Leonard JL, Davis PJ. Molecular aspects of thyroid hormone actions. Endocr Rev. 2010;31:139–70. https://doi.org/10.1210/er.2009-0007.
3. Cioffi F, Giacco A, Goglia F, Silvestri E. Bioenergetic aspects of mitochondrial actions of thyroid hormones. Cells. 2022;11:997. https://doi.org/10.3390/cells11060997.
4. Biondi B, Cooper DS. The clinical significance of subclinical thyroid dysfunction. Endocr Rev. 2008;29:76–131. https://doi.org/10.1210/er.2006-0043.
5. Chaker L, Bianco AC, Jonklaas J, Peeters RP. Hypothyroidism. Lancet. 2017;390:1550–62. https://doi.org/10.1016/S0140-6736(17)30703-1.
6. Jansen HI, Boelen A, Heijboer AC, Bruinstroop E, Fliers E. Hypothyroidism: the difficulty in attributing symptoms to their underlying cause. Front Endocrinol (Lausanne). 2023;14:1130661. https://doi.org/10.3389/fendo.2023.1130661.
7. Jonklaas J, Bianco AC, Bauer AJ, Burman KD, Cappola AR, Celi FS, Cooper DS, Kim BW, Peeters RP, Rosenthal MS, Sawka AM. Guidelines for the treatment of hypothyroidism: prepared by the American Thyroid Association task force on thyroid hormone replacement. Thyroid. 2014;24:1670–751. https://doi.org/10.1089/thy.2014.0028.
8. Vanderpump MP, Tunbridge WM, French JM, Appleton D, Bates DM, Clark F, Grimley Evans J, Hasan DM, Rodgers H, Tunbridge F. The incidence of thyroid disorders in the community: a twenty-year follow-up of the Whickham survey. Clin Endocrinol. 1995;43:55–68. https://doi.org/10.1111/j.1365-2265.1995.tb01894.x.
9. Canaris GJ, Manowitz NR. The Colorado thyroid disease prevalence study. Arch Intern Med. 2000;160:526–34. https://doi.org/10.1001/archinte.160.4.526.
10. Flynn RWV, Macdonald TM, Morris AD, Jung RT, Leese GP. The thyroid epidemiology, audit, and research study: thyroid dysfunction in the general population. J Clin Endocrinol Metab. 2004;89:3879–84. https://doi.org/10.1210/jc.2003-032089.
11. Garmendia Madariaga A, Santos Palacios S, Guillén-Grima F, Galofré JC. The incidence and prevalence of thyroid dysfunction in Europe: a meta-analysis. J Clin Endocrinol Metab. 2014;99:923–31. https://doi.org/10.1210/jc.2013-2409.
12. Valdés S, Maldonado-Araque C, Lago-Sampedro A, Lillo JA, Garcia-Fuentes E, Perez-Valero V, Gutierrez-Repiso C, Ocon-Sanchez P, Goday A, Urrutia I, Peláez L, Calle-Pascual A, Bordiú E, Castaño L, Castell C, Delgado E, Menendez E, Franch J, Gaztambide S, Girbés J, Ortega E, Lopez-Alba A, Chaves FJ, Vendrell J, Chacón MR, Soriguer F, Rojo-Martínez G. Population-based national prevalence of thyroid dysfunction in Spain and associated factors: diabetes study. Thyroid. 2017;27:156–66. https://doi.org/10.1089/thy.2016.0353.
13. Taylor PN, Albrecht D, Scholz A, Gutierrez-Buey G, Lazarus JH, Dayan CM, Okosieme OE. Global epidemiology of hyperthyroidism and hypothyroidism. Nat Rev Endocrinol. 2018;14:301–16. https://doi.org/10.1038/nrendo.2018.18.
14. Wouters HJCM, Slagter SN, Muller Kobold AC, Van Der Klauw MM, Wolffenbuttel BHR. Epidemiology of thyroid disorders in the lifelines cohort study (The Netherlands). PLoS One. 2020;15:e0242795. https://doi.org/10.1371/journal.pone.0242795.
15. Chaker L, Razvi S, Bensenor IM, Azizi F, Pearce EN, Peeters RP. Hypothyroidism. Natl Rev. 2022;8:30. https://doi.org/10.1038/s41572-022-00357-7.
16. Wyne KL, Nair L, Schneiderman CP, Pinsky B, Antunez Flores O, Guo D, Barger B, Tessnow AH. Hypothyroidism prevalence in the United States: a retrospective study combining national health and nutrition examination survey and claims data, 2009-2019. J Endocr Soc. 2022;7:bvac172. https://doi.org/10.1210/jendso/bvac172.
17. Johannesen HL, Veyhe AS, Andreassen J, Weihe P, Strøm M, Andorsdóttir G, Rasmussen AK, Feldt-Rasmussen U, Carlé A, Andersen S. A nationwide registry-based observational study of thyroid disease incidence in the Faroe Islands. Clin Endocrinol. 2024;100(6):575–84. https://doi.org/10.1111/cen.15050.

18. Beck-Peccoz P, Rodari G, Giavoli C, Lania A. Central hypothyroidism—a neglected thyroid disorder. Nat Rev Endocrinol. 2017;13:588–98. https://doi.org/10.1038/nrendo.2017.47.
19. Hoermann R, Midgley JEM, Larisch R, Dietrich JW. Relational stability in the expression of normality, variation, and control of thyroid function. Front Endocrinol (Lausanne). 2016;7:142. https://doi.org/10.3389/fendo.2016.00142.
20. Pappa T, Refetoff S. Resistance to thyroid hormone beta: a focused review. Front Endocrinol (Lausanne). 2021;12:656551. https://doi.org/10.3389/fendo.2021.656551.
21. Hashimoto H. Zur Kenntnis der lymphomatösen Veränderung der Schilddrüse (struma lymphomatosda). Arch klin Chir (Berlin). 1912;97:219–50.
22. Bergemann N, Jonsdottir B, Nilsson A-L, Lantz M, Lind A. Prevalence of thyroid peroxidase and thyroglobulin autoantibodies in the Swedish population. Exp Clin Endocrinol Diabetes. 2023;131:456–62. https://doi.org/10.1055/a-2096-9641.
23. Ziaka M, Exadaktylos A. Insights into sars-cov-2-associated subacute thyroiditis: from infection to vaccine. Virol J. 2023;20:132. https://doi.org/10.1186/s12985-023-02103-1.
24. Lauretta R, Sansone A, Sansone M, Romanelli F, Appetecchia M. Endocrine disrupting chemicals: effects on endocrine glands. Front Endocrinol (Lausanne). 2019;10:178. https://doi.org/10.3389/fendo.2019.00178.
25. Burman KD, Baker JR Jr. Immune mechanisms in Graves' disease. Endocr Rev. 1985;6:183–232.
26. Weetman AP. Grave's disease 1835-2002. Horm Res. 2003;59(Suppl 1):114–8. https://doi.org/10.1159/000067837.
27. Antonelli A, Ferrari SM, Corrado A, Di Domenicantonio A, Fallahi P. Autoimmune thyroid disorders. Autoimmun Rev. 2015;14:174–80. https://doi.org/10.1016/j.autrev.2014.10.016.
28. Klubo-Gwiezdzinska J, Wartofsky L. Hashimoto thyroiditis: an evidence-based guide: etiology, diagnosis and treatment. Pol Arch Intern Med. 2022;132:16222.
29. Milo T, Korem Kohanim Y, Toledano Y, Alon U. Autoimmune thyroid diseases as a cost of physiological autoimmune surveillance. Trends Immunol. 2023;44(5):365–71. https://doi.org/10.1016/j.it.2023.03.007.
30. Boelaert K, Newby PR, Simmonds MJ, Holder RL, Carr-Smith JD, Heward JM, Manji N, Allahabadia A, Armitage M, Chatterjee KV, Lazarus JH, Pearce SH, Vaidya B, Gough SC, Franklyn JA. Prevalence and relative risk of other autoimmune diseases in subjects with autoimmune thyroid disease. Am J Med. 2010;123(183):e1–9. https://doi.org/10.1016/j.amjmed.2009.06.030.
31. Wiersinga WM, Poppe KG, Effraimidis G. Hyperthyroidism: etiology, pathogenesis, diagnosis, management, complications, and prognosis. Lancet Diabetes Endocrinol. 2023;11:282–98. https://doi.org/10.1016/S2213-8587(23)00005-0.
32. Costagliola S, Morgenthaler NG, Hoermann R, Badenhoop K, Struck J, Freitag D, Poertl S, Weglöhner W, Hollidt JM, Quadbeck B, Dumont JE, Schumm-Draeger PM, Bergmann A, Mann K, Vassart G, Usadel KH. Second generation assay for thyrotropin receptor antibodies has superior diagnostic sensitivity for Graves' disease. J Clin Endocrinol Metab. 1999;84:90–7. https://doi.org/10.1210/jcem.84.1.5415.
33. Hoermann R, Midgley JEM, Larisch R, Dietrich JW. Homeostatic control of the thyroid-pituitary axis: perspectives for diagnosis and treatment. Front Endocrinol (Lausanne). 2015;6:177. https://doi.org/10.3389/fendo.2015.00177.
34. Weetman AP. An update on the pathogenesis of Hashimoto's thyroiditis. J Endocrinol Investig. 2021;44:883–90. https://doi.org/10.1007/s40618-020-01477-1.
35. Vassart G, Dumont JE. The thyrotropin receptor and the regulation of thyrocyte function and growth. Endocr Rev. 1992;13:596–611. https://doi.org/10.1210/edrv-13-3-596.
36. Korem Kohanim Y, Milo T, Raz M, Karin O, Bar A, Mayo A, Mendelson Cohen N, Toledano Y, Alon U. Dynamics of thyroid diseases and thyroid-axis gland masses. Mol Syst Biol. 2022;18:e10919. https://doi.org/10.15252/msb.202210919.
37. Raz M, Milo T, Glass DS, Mayo A, Alon U. Endocrine gland size is proportional to its target tissue size. iScience. 2024;27(9):110625. https://doi.org/10.1016/j.isci.2024.110625.

38. Dugrillon A, Bechtner G, Uedelhoven WM, Weber PC, Gärtner R. Evidence that an iodolactone mediates the inhibitory effect of iodide on thyroid cell proliferation but not on adenosine 3′,5′-monophosphate formation. Endocrinology. 1990;127:337–43. https://doi.org/10.1210/endo-127-1-337.
39. Tendler A, Bar A, Mendelsohn-Cohen N, Karin O, Korem Kohanim Y, Maimon L, Milo T, Raz M, Mayo A, Tanay A, Alon U. Hormone seasonality in medical records suggests circannual endocrine circuits. Proc Natl Acad Sci USA. 2021;118(7):e2003926118. https://doi.org/10.1073/pnas.2003926118.
40. Yamada S, Horiguchi K, Akuzawa M, Sakamaki K, Shimomura Y, Kobayashi I, Andou Y, Yamada M. Seasonal variation in thyroid function in over 7,000 healthy subjects in an iodine-sufficient area and literature review. J Endocr Soc. 2022;6:bvac054. https://doi.org/10.1210/jendso/bvac054.
41. Leow MKS. A review of the phenomenon of hysteresis in the hypothalamus-pituitary-thyroid axis. Front Endocrinol (Lausanne). 2016;7:64. https://doi.org/10.3389/fendo.2016.00064.
42. Fitzgerald SP, Bean NG, Falhammar H, Hoermann R. Physiological linkage of thyroid and pituitary sensitivities. Endocrine. 2023;79:143–51. https://doi.org/10.1007/s12020-022-03184-8.
43. Fitzgerald SP, Bean NG, Falhammar H, Hoermann R, Korem Kohanim Y, Pohlabeln H, Grote Beverborg N, Tomassetti S. Population data evidence of interdependence of the limbs of hormonal feedback loops. J Endocrinol. 2024;262:e230384. https://doi.org/10.1530/JOE-23-0384.
44. Hoermann R, Schumm-Draeger PM, Rehbach K, Mann K. Asialoagalacto-human chorionic gonadotropin, a carbohydrate-modified variant of human chorionic gonadotropin, antagonizes the stimulatory actions of bovine thyroid-stimulating hormone on thyroid function and hla-dr expression in human thyroid in vitro and in vivo. J Clin Invest. 1991;88:1947–54. https://doi.org/10.1172/JCI115519.
45. Hoermann R, Schumm-Draeger PM, Mann K. Inhibition of functional and immunological responses to thyroid-stimulating antibodies from patients with Graves' disease by blockade of the thyrotropin receptor. Thyroid. 1993;3:273–8. https://doi.org/10.1089/thy.1993.3.273.
46. Hoermann R, Spitzweg C, Poertl S, Mann K, Heufelder AE, Schumm-Draeger PM. Regulation of intercellular adhesion molecule-1 expression in human thyroid cells in vitro and human thyroid tissue transplanted to the nude mouse in vivo: role of Graves' immunoglobulins and human thyrotropin receptor. J Clin Endocrinol Metab. 1997;82:2048–55. https://doi.org/10.1210/jcem.82.7.4058.
47. Sarkar R, Bolel P, Kapoor A, Eliseeva E, Dulcey AE, Templin JS, Wang AQ, Xu X, Southall N, Klubo-Gwiezdzinska J, Neumann S, Marugan JJ, Gershengorn MC. An orally efficacious thyrotropin receptor ligand inhibits growth and metastatic activity of thyroid cancers. J Clin Endocrinol Metab. 2024;109:2306–16. https://doi.org/10.1210/clinem/dgae114.
48. Caturegli P, De Remigis A, Rose NR. Hashimoto thyroiditis: clinical and diagnostic criteria. Autoimmun Rev. 2014;13:391–7. https://doi.org/10.1016/j.autrev.2014.01.007.
49. Quadbeck B, Eckstein AK, Tews S, Walz M, Hoermann R, Mann K, Gieseler R. Maturation of thyroidal dendritic cells in Graves' disease. Scand J Immunol. 2002;55:612–20. https://doi.org/10.1046/j.1365-3083.2002.01066.x.
50. Eckstein A, Quadbeck B, Mueller G, Rettenmeier AW, Hoermann R, Mann K, Steuhl P, Esser J. Impact of smoking on the response to treatment of thyroid associated ophthalmopathy. Br J Ophthalmol. 2003;87:773–6. https://doi.org/10.1136/bjo.87.6.773.
51. Abu Rached N, Dietrich JW, Ocker L, Quast DR, Scheel C, Gambichler T, Bechara FG. Primary thyroid dysfunction is prevalent in hidradenitis suppurativa and marked by a signature of hypothyroid Graves' disease: a case–control study. J Clin Med. 2023;12:7490. https://doi.org/10.3390/jcm12237490.
52. Lebel Y, Milo T, Bar A, Mayo A, Alon U. Excitable dynamics of flares and relapses in autoimmune diseases. iScience. 2023;26:108084. https://doi.org/10.1016/j.isci.2023.108084.
53. Mathiopoulou M, Engel-Bicik I. Hyperthyroidism in 2 forms: the Marine-Lenhart syndrome. Endocr Abstr. 2023;93:OC42. https://doi.org/10.1530/endoabs.93.oc42.

Chapter 2
The Concept of Relational Stability

Rudolf Hoermann and Johannes W. Dietrich

A multitude of physiological reactions and metabolic functions in the human body depend on the actions of thyroid hormones. For their proper functioning thyroid hormone concentrations must be kept in a narrow range both over long periods of time and during varying internal changes and imposed external conditions [1]. Tight control of circulating thyroid hormone concentrations is therefore a primary goal for attaining and maintaining a state of thyroid health [2]. This, in turn, creates a state of internal stability for the many biochemical reactions and metabolic processes that work at a narrow temperature optimum in the mammalian organism. Gaining control over energy expenditure independently of environmental short-term supply through the internal working of the thyroid system offers major systemic advantages [3]. This is a key role for the thyroid system which involves the hypothalamic–pituitary–thyroid axis regulation [1, 4]. A system failure may lead to thyroid dysfunction and hypothyroidism.

R. Hoermann (✉)
Yandina, QLD, Australia

Department of General Internal Medicine, Gastroenterology and Endocrinology, [Retired] Klinikum Lüdenscheid, Lüdenscheid, Germany
e-mail: rudolf.hoermann@gmail.com

J. W. Dietrich
Diabetes, Endocrinology and Metabolism Section, Department of Medicine, St. Josef-Hospital, Ruhr University Hospitals, Bochum, Germany

Centre for Diabetes Technology (ZDT), Catholic Hospitals Bochum, Bochum, Germany

Centre for Rare Endocrine Diseases (ZSEK), Ruhr Center for Rare Diseases (CeSER), Ruhr University of Bochum and Witten/Herdecke University, Bochum, Germany

Centre for Thyroid Medicine (ZSM), Ruhr University of Bochum, Bochum, Germany
e-mail: johannes.dietrich@ruhr-uni-bochum.de

R. Hoermann, J. W. Dietrich (eds.), *Hypothyroidism*,
https://doi.org/10.1007/978-981-96-3682-2_2

This type of regulatory control has been generally expressed by the concept of homeostasis [5–10]. Here, we are particularly interested in the homeostasis (stability) of FT3, the biologically active thyroid hormone, as a systemic goal of hypothalamic–pituitary–thyroid regulation (Chap. 5). This is attained through *relational stability* between the three hormones TSH, FT4 and FT3, where, as explained below, the actions of TSH and FT4 oppose each other but combine to support FT3 homeostasis.

Homeostasis by definition includes a self-regulating process which enables the organism to maintain a state of internal stability while adjusting, at the same time, to changing external conditions. In essence, this is a dynamic process that can change internal conditions as required to survive external challenges [9]. To this end, the homeostatic regulation of thyroid hormones extends beyond a single negative feedback loop between the pituitary hormone TSH and the main thyroid hormone FT4, as discussed in detail later (Chap. 5). Rather it is described through a complex network of multiple feedback and feed-forward limbs, interacting in a reciprocal mode of top–down and bottom–up control [4].

A combined view of all thyroid parameters and their interrelationships may therefore provide a more comprehensive picture, compared to the application of statistically derived separate reference intervals for each thyroid parameter [4]. Accordingly, due to their interdependence, the biological normality of "thyroid health" in an individual is more narrowly defined as a perceived optimal state and corresponding appropriate level of each hormone, rather than assuming a satisfactory outcome using a much wider reference range in a population [11, 12]. Appropriately, when measuring the three main thyroid hormones, TSH, FT4 and FT3, clinicians should not view these parameters independently of each other, rather consider their integrated systemic roles and interdependent homeostatically regulated equilibrium [2, 13]. This is what we termed "relational stability" [2]. The very idea of balance and harmony as necessary conditions for health and the survival of living organisms dates back to the fourth century BC and the Greek philosopher Empedocles [14].

The concept of relational stability is supported by recent advances in our understanding of system regulation and system endocrinology [4, 15–17]. The concept describes the adaptive and range-dependent interrelations between the parameters that combine to support homeostasis and system stability [2]. Rather than univariate expression of normality in a single component, an interpretation of the joint expression of all thyroid parameters and their interrelationships provides a more accurate picture of the situational relevance of the respective adaptive homeostatic equilibria between TSH and thyroid hormones [2]. "Disruption of homeostatic mechanisms" is what leads to disease according to Billman [9], and effective therapy must be directed towards "re-establishing these homeostatic conditions" [9].

We will examine the concept using two prevalent clinical constellations, i.e. that of subclinical hypothyroidism and athyroidism (LT4-treated patients without a thyroid).

Subclinical hypothyroidism, as defined by guidelines [18], remains an ambiguous diagnosis because a moderately raised TSH could either signal successful homeostatic adaptation or indicate a failed attempt at restoration of euthyroidism [19]. Supporting the former view, the majority of clinical studies showed no adverse outcomes for mortality, cardiovascular events, fracture risk or cognitive impairment in association with mildly elevated TSH levels (5–10 mIU/l) per se [20, 21]. However, a recent meta-analysis observed an increased risk for sudden cardiac death in subclinical hypothyroidism. It remains unclear if the results are confounded by stress-related TSH elevation or if they mirror stimulated T3 formation as explained in detail below [22].

At the onset of thyroid gland failure with diminishing thyroid hormone supply following transient or less severe disruptions, relational stability appears to be an effective early line of defence against such phenomena and the development of hypothyroidism [2] (Fig. 2.1). Disease manifestation becomes dependent on the progressive alteration in the controlling interplay between TSH, FT4 and FT3 across the range. If left uncorrected, the disruption of homeostatic mechanisms may lead to disease [9]. As the system seeks to respond in a preventive and proactive way by activating corrective mechanisms from the onset of thyroid capacity stress, maintenance of FT3 homeostatic positions takes priority over set point fixation in expressing the TSH–FT4–FT3 relationship [2] (Fig. 2.1). The system response consequently aims to increase global deiodinase activity and direct T3 secretion as thyroidal T4 production declines in early thyroid failure [15, 23]. Of note, to enable homeostasis of FT3, the latter becomes uncorrelated from TSH and FT4 concentrations in the euthyroid range [24]. The mechanisms of the supportive actions of TSH on FT3 homeostasis are detailed in Chap. 5.

Recent studies confirmed more broadly that, contrary to a widely held belief [18], TSH and FT4 may not be accurate surrogates of FT3 due to "an unappreciated complexity of the HPT-axis signaling cascade" [25]. Furthermore, Lawton et al. found that "subclinical variation in the HPT-axis effector hormone T3 is an

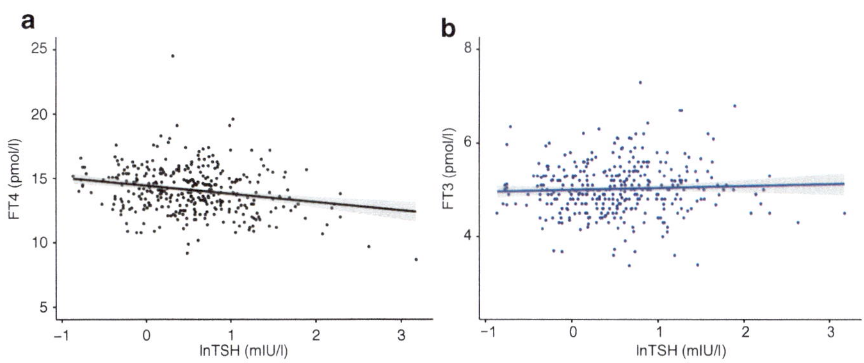

Fig. 2.1 Relational stability between TSH, FT4 and FT3 and preservation of FT3 homeostasis As TSH and FT4 move in opposite directions in euthyroid and subclinically hypothyroid patients (**a**), FT3 concentrations do not parallel the decline of FT4 concentrations but remain homeostatically controlled and stable over a wide range of TSH values (**b**) [2]. (Data are from a clinical study [23])

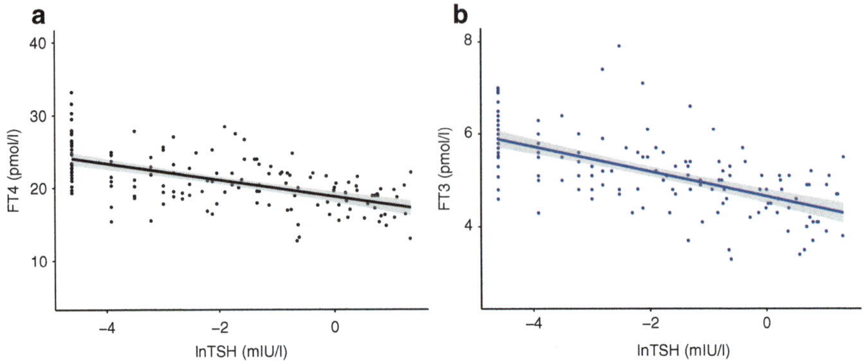

Fig. 2.2 Absence of relational stability and loss of FT3 homeostasis in athyreotic LT4-treated patients
Unlike in the healthy condition and subclinical hypothyroidism, as shown in Fig. 2.1 above, FT3 homeostasis is broken in the absence of a functioning thyroid gland [2]. It is no longer preserved and protected by TSH and FT4 (**a**). Rather FT3 levels are now correlated with both FT4 and TSH concentrations (**b**). (Data are from a clinical study [24])

important and overlooked factor linking socio-economic forces, human biology, and aging" [25].

In a study on LT4-treated athyreotic patients after thyroidectomy mainly due to thyroid cancer, we found the corrective actions of the TSH-FT3 shunt (feed-forward) within the thyroid gland to be no longer operative [2]. As a consequence, alterations in the interlocking relationships and governing equilibria arise between TSH, FT4 and FT3 levels, and FT3 homeostasis breaks down [2]. This, in turn, renders the association of FT3 concentrations with TSH levels unbalanced and homeostatically unstable, resulting in a progressive disjoint between TSH and FT3 in these patients (Fig. 2.2). Clinically, this has been shown to lead to wide variations in the biochemical and symptomatic responses in patients to LT4 treatment [26]. As a serious consequence, many patients may thus continue to suffer from persisting clinical symptoms even after apparently "normalising" their TSH level (bringing it into the reference range) with LT4 treatment [12]. Even the probability of TSH suppression is higher than that of FT3 normalisation above mid-range [26]. Implications for patient treatment will be considered in more detail in other chapters.

In conclusion, the concept of relational stability strongly argues against the predominant position that has been given to TSH [18], suggesting that parameters other than TSH should be assigned a more defining role in the diagnosis and treatment of thyroid health and disease including both thyroid hormones FT4 and FT3 and their ratios. This adds to other calls for a critical re-analysis of the current preference for TSH levels in the assessment of the thyroid state of the peripheral tissues [25, 27].

In particular, the interrelations between thyroid hormones, such as FT3–FT4 ratio or calculated SPINA step-up deiodinase activity (SPINA-GD), and other structural thyroid parameters, such as estimated functional thyroid capacity (SPINA-GT) and set point reconstruction, have emerged as research tools to develop novel clinically useful algorithms [28] (Sect. 10.3). New markers of tissue responses to thyroid hormones including metabolic profiling should also be useful and worth exploring [29, 30].

In the following chapters, we will first review the foundations of thyroid physiology before revisiting the regulation of thyroid hormones in more detail.

References

1. Hoermann R, Midgley JEM, Larisch R, Dietrich JW. Homeostatic control of the thyroid-pituitary axis: perspectives for diagnosis and treatment. Front Endocrinol (Lausanne). 2015;6:177. https://doi.org/10.3389/fendo.2015.00177.
2. Hoermann R, Midgley JEM, Larisch R, Dietrich JW. Relational stability in the expression of normality, variation, and control of thyroid function. Front Endocrinol (Lausanne). 2016;7:142. https://doi.org/10.3389/fendo.2016.00142.
3. Suarez R. The biology of energy expenditure. J Exp Biol. 2011;214:163–3. https://doi.org/10.1242/jeb.053835.
4. Hoermann R, Pekker M, Midgley JEM, Larisch R, Dietrich JW. Principles of endocrine regulation: reconciling tensions between robustness in performance and adaptation to change. Front Endocrinol (Lausanne). 2022;13:825107. https://doi.org/10.3389/fendo.2022.825107.
5. Cannon WB, Rosenberg CE. Homeostasis. The wisdom of the body. New York: Norton; 1932.
6. Modell H, Cliff W, Michael J, Mcfarland J, Wenderoth MP, Wright A. A physiologist's view of homeostasis. Adv Physiol Educ. 2015;39:259–66. https://doi.org/10.1152/advan.00107.2015.
7. Reed M, Best J, Golubitsky M, Stewart I, Nijhout HF. Analysis of homeostatic mechanisms in biochemical networks. Bull Math Biol. 2017;79:2534–57. https://doi.org/10.1007/s11538-017-0340-z.
8. Golubitsky M, Stewart I, Antoneli F, Huang Z, Wang Y. Input-output networks, singularity theory, and homeostasis. Advances in dynamics, optimization and computation. In: Proceedings of the workshop on dynamics, optimization and computation held in honor of the 60th birthday of Michael Dellnitz; 2020. p. 31–65. https://doi.org/10.1007/978-3-030-51264-4_2.
9. Billman GE. Homeostasis: the underappreciated and far too often ignored central organizing principle of physiology. Front Physiol. 2020;11:200. https://doi.org/10.3389/fphys.2020.00200.
10. Goldstein DS. Stress and the "extended" autonomic system. Auton Neurosci. 2021;236:102889. https://doi.org/10.1016/j.autneu.2021.102889.
11. Andersen S, Pedersen KM, Bruun NH, Laurberg P. Narrow individual variations in serum T4 and T3 in normal subjects: a clue to the understanding of subclinical thyroid disease. J Clin Endocrinol Metal. 2002;87:1068–72. https://doi.org/10.1210/jcem.87.3.8165.
12. Hoermann R, Midgley JEM, Larisch R, Dietrich JW. Functional and symptomatic individuality in the response to levothyroxine treatment. Front Endocrinol (Lausanne). 2019;10:664. https://doi.org/10.3389/fendo.2019.00664.
13. Fitzgerald SP, Bean NG, Falhammar H, Hoermann R. Physiological linkage of thyroid and pituitary sensitivities. Endocrine. 2023;79:143–51. https://doi.org/10.1007/s12020-022-03184-8.
14. Stavros BJ. Empedocles and neurosciences. Encephalos. 2014;51:66–78.
15. Hoermann R, Pekker MJ, Midgley JEM, Dietrich JW. The role of supporting and disruptive mechanisms of FT3 homeostasis in regulating the hypothalamic-pituitary-thyroid axis. Ther Adv Endocrinol Metab. 2023;14:20420188231158163. https://doi.org/10.1177/20420188231158163.
16. Raz M, Milo T, Glass DS, Mayo A, Alon U. Endocrine gland size is proportional to its target tissue size. iScience. 2024;27(9):110625. https://doi.org/10.1016/j.isci.2024.110625.

17. Raz M, Glass DS, Milo T, Kohanim YK, Karin O, Tendler A, Mayo A, Alon U. Unifying regulatory motifs in endocrine circuits. bioRxiv. 2024; https://doi.org/10.1101/2024.08.06.606903.
18. Jonklaas J, Bianco AC, Bauer AJ, Burman KD, Cappola AR, Celi FS, Cooper DS, Kim BW, Peeters RP, Rosenthal MS, Sawka AM. Guidelines for the treatment of hypothyroidism: prepared by the American Thyroid Association task force on thyroid hormone replacement. Thyroid. 2014;24:1670–751. https://doi.org/10.1089/thy.2014.0028.
19. Dietrich JW, Hoermann R, Midgley JEM, Bergen F, Müller P. The two faces of janus: why thyrotropin as a cardiovascular risk factor may be an ambiguous target. Front Endocrinol (Lausanne). 2020;11:829. https://doi.org/10.3389/fendo.2020.542710.
20. Stott DJ, Rodondi N, Kearney PM, Ford I, Westendorp RGJ, Mooijaart SP, Sattar N, Aubert CE, Aujesky D, Bauer DC, Baumgartner C, Blum MR, Browne JP, Byrne S, Collet TH, Dekkers OM, Den Elzen WPJ, Du Puy RS, Ellis G, Feller M, Floriani C, Hendry K, Hurley C, Jukema JW, Kean S, Kelly M, Krebs D, Langhorne P, Mccarthy G, Mccarthy V, Mcconnachie A, Mcdade M, Messow M, O'flynn A, O'riordan D, Poortvliet RKE, Quinn TJ, Russell A, Sinnott C, Smit JWA, Van Dorland HA, Walsh KA, Walsh EK, Watt T, Wilson R, Gussekloo J, Trust SG. Thyroid hormone therapy for older adults with subclinical hypothyroidism. N Engl J Med. 2017;376:2534–44. https://doi.org/10.1056/NEJMoa1603825.
21. Biondi B, Cappola AR, Cooper DS. Subclinical hypothyroidism: a review. JAMA. 2019;322:153–60. https://doi.org/10.1001/jama.2019.9052.
22. Müller P, Leow MK, Dietrich JW. Minor perturbations of thyroid homeostasis and major cardiovascular endpoints-Physiological mechanisms and clinical evidence. Front Cardiovasc Med. 2022;9:942971. https://doi.org/10.3389/fcvm.2022.942971. PMID: 36046184; PMCID: PMC9420854
23. Hoermann R, Midgley JEM, Larisch R, Dietrich JW. Relational stability of thyroid hormones in euthyroid subjects and patients with autoimmune thyroid disease. Eur Thyroid J. 2016;5:171–9. https://doi.org/10.1159/000447967.
24. Hoermann R, Midgley JEM, Giacobino A, Eckl WA, Wahl HG, Dietrich JW, Larisch R. Homeostatic equilibria between free thyroid hormones and pituitary thyrotropin are modulated by various influences including age, body mass index and treatment. Clin Endocrinol. 2014;81:907–15. https://doi.org/10.1111/cen.12527.
25. Lawton RI, Sabatini BL, Hochbaum DR. Longevity, demographic characteristics, and socio-economic status are linked to triiodothyronine levels in the general population. Proc Natl Acad Sci USA. 2024;121(2):e2308652121. https://doi.org/10.1073/pnas.2308652121.
26. Midgley JEM, Larisch R, Dietrich JW, Hoermann R. Variation in the biochemical response to L-thyroxine therapy and relationship with peripheral thyroid hormone conversion efficiency. Endocr Connect. 2015;4:196–205. https://doi.org/10.1530/EC-15-0056.
27. Fitzgerald SP, Bean NG, Hennessey JV, Falhammar H. Thyroid testing paradigm switch from thyrotropin to thyroid hormones-future directions and opportunities in clinical medicine and research. Endocrine. 2021;74:285–9. https://doi.org/10.1007/s12020-021-02851-6.
28. Dietrich JW, Landgrafe-Mende G, Wiora E, Chatzitomaris A, Klein HH, Midgley JEM, Hoermann R. Calculated parameters of thyroid homeostasis: emerging tools for differential diagnosis and clinical research. Front Endocrinol (Lausanne). 2016;7:57. https://doi.org/10.3389/fendo.2016.00057.
29. Massolt ET, Meima ME, Swagemakers SMA, Leeuwenburgh S, Van Den Hout-Van Vroonhoven MCGM, Brigante G, Kam BLR, Van Der Spek PJ, Van Ijcken WFJ, Visser TJ, Peeters RP, Visser WE. Thyroid state regulates gene expression in human whole blood. J Clin Endocrinol Metab. 2018;103:169–78. https://doi.org/10.1210/jc.2017-01144.
30. Jaber MA, Benabdelkamel H, Dahabiyeh LA, Masood A, Almalki RH, Musambil M, Alfadda AA, Abdel Rahman AM. The metabolomics approach revealed a distinctive metabolomics pattern associated with hyperthyroidism treatment. Front Endocrinol (Lausanne). 2022;13:1050201. https://doi.org/10.3389/fendo.2022.1050201.

Chapter 3
Thyroid Physiology

Rudolf Hoermann and Johannes W. Dietrich

Thyroid hormones are members of the large family of iodothyronines and the even larger family of thyronine derivatives, which includes iodothyroacetates and thyronamines as well.

During evolution, many living organisms including plants, animals and humans developed the capability to bind the inorganic trace element iodine to proteins [1]. Along with these evolutionary developments, a specialised organ emerged for the storage of both iodine and thyroid hormones to facilitate the complex pathway from iodine uptake, accumulation, storage, organification and thyroid hormone synthesis and on-demand secretion. Of note, unlike other endocrine organs, the thyroid stores pre-synthesised hormones in its follicles for fast release upon demand. In humans, the production of iodothyronines mainly comprises two distinct hormones, namely *thyroxine* (*T4*) and *triiodothyronine* (*T3*) [2] (Fig. 3.1).

Notably, the thyroid is not unique in being able to accumulate iodine, but it is the only organ capable of synthesising both T4 and T3. Whilst other organs than the

R. Hoermann (✉)
Yandina, QLD, Australia

Department of General Internal Medicine, Gastroenterology and Endocrinology,
[Retired] Klinikum Lüdenscheid, Lüdenscheid, Germany
e-mail: rudolf.hoermann@gmail.com

J. W. Dietrich
Diabetes, Endocrinology and Metabolism Section, Department of Medicine,
St. Josef-Hospital, Ruhr University Hospitals, Bochum, Germany

Centre for Diabetes Technology (ZDT), Catholic Hospitals Bochum, Bochum, Germany

Centre for Rare Endocrine Diseases (ZSEK), Ruhr Center for Rare Diseases (CeSER),
Ruhr University of Bochum and Witten/Herdecke University, Bochum, Germany

Centre for Thyroid Medicine (ZSM), Ruhr University of Bochum, Bochum, Germany
e-mail: johannes.dietrich@ruhr-uni-bochum.de

R. Hoermann, J. W. Dietrich (eds.), *Hypothyroidism*,
https://doi.org/10.1007/978-981-96-3682-2_3

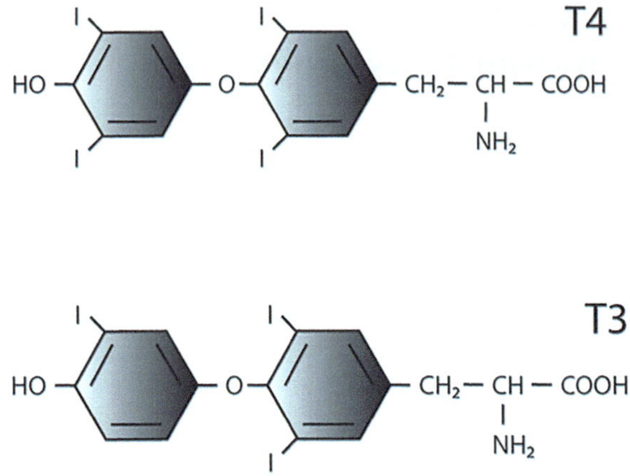

Fig. 3.1 Biochemical structure of the main thyroid hormones T4 and T3

thyroid gland are unable to produce T4, they are able to generate T3 from T4 via enzymatic deiodination [3] (see Sect. 3.5). Owing to their fundamental importance for metabolic control, the synthesis and release of thyroid hormones is a tightly regulated physiological process [4]. Apart from T4 and T3, termed the classical thyroid hormones, numerous non-classical thyroid hormones, such as *reverse triiodothyronine (rT3), 3,5-diiodothyronine* (3,5-*T2*), *iodothyroacetates* and *thyronamines,* have been recognised to play more active physiological roles than previously assumed [5–11].

3.1 Iodine and Thyroid Hormone Metabolism

The influence of nutritional factors, particularly *iodine* and *selenium*, on thyroid function and its diseases has long been recognised (Sect. 11.7). The therapeutic use of iodine-rich sea weed dates back to ancient China about 3000 years BC and that of iodine salt from the lower Nile to ancient Egypt [12]. In Europe, alimentary iodine deficiency has been a consequence of the last Ice Age where movements of glaciers leached out this mineral from the soil into the sea. In modern times, many countries have introduced iodine monitoring and supplementing programmes to successfully combat the serious consequences of iodine deficiency disorders [13]. Severe iodine deficiency could thereby be almost completely eliminated as a cause of hypothyroidism. Excessive iodine intake can also cause hypothyroidism in susceptible individuals and exacerbate thyroid autoimmune disease. Lugol's solution is a medically used thyroid hormone release blocker.

Naturally, the trace element iodine is ingested with food and to a lesser extent with drinking water. It is readily absorbed as iodide in the small intestine (Fig. 3.2). Approximately 60% is cleared from the circulation by the kidneys, and 40% is taken up by the thyroid. Renal iodine excretion reflects the nutritional supply of the

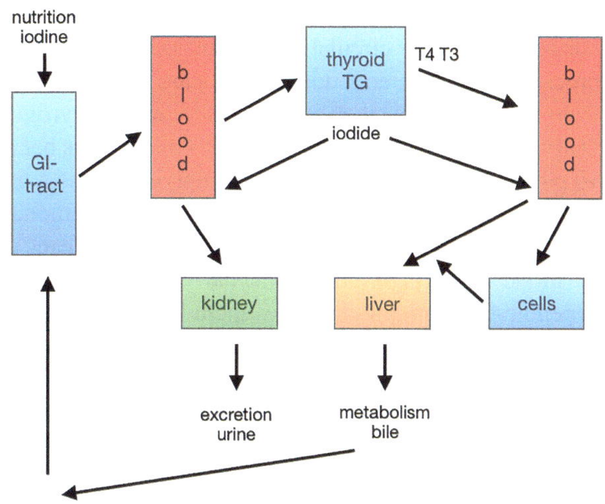

Fig. 3.2 Scheme of iodine metabolism
Refer to text for a detailed description*GI-tract* gastrointestinal tract, *TG* thyroglobulin

element and may therefore be used as a marker of alimentary iodine sufficiency or deficiency in population screening. Due to considerable variations, this is less useful for individual screening. Thyroidal iodine uptake from the circulation against an adverse gradient is an active, energy-consuming, specific and controlled process. It is facilitated by an iodide pump, the sodium iodide symporter [14, 15]. Two important regulators of the activity of the pump are the intrathyroidal iodide content and the pituitary hormone TSH. The physiological daily iodine intake amounts to approximately 100–150 μg, with an adaptable intrathyroidal concentration factor of 20–50. Thyroid hormone secretion can be maintained up to a critical iodine deficit by increasing the activity of the iodide symporter. Due to its intrathyroidal accumulation, the biological effects of iodine outlast its half-life in the circulation, thereby buffering against daily variations in alimentary iodine supply, but not compensating for a chronic deficiency (<100 μg/day). In the event of acute iodine excess, iodine uptake is shut down by the healthy thyroid by two distinct intrathyroidal feed-forward and feedback mechanisms referred to as the Plummer and the Wolff-Chaikoff effect, but not so in pathological conditions, particularly thyroid autonomy [16].

At the apical membrane of the thyroid follicular cell iodide is oxidised to iodine and incorporated into a tyrosyl residue of the thyroglobulin (Tg) molecule. This process of iodine organification is mediated by a specific enzyme thyroid peroxidase (TPO). The precursors 3-monotyrosine (MIT) and 3,5-diiodothyrosine (DIT) are then joined to synthesise the two thyroid hormones triiodothyronine (T3) and thyroxine (T4) [17]. Of note, thyroidal T3 can be derived by two ways, namely through de-novo synthesis and 5-monodeiodination of T4. The amount of T3 that is produced relative to that of T4 is directly correlated to the availability of iodine, increasing the FT3–FT4 ratio in the event of iodine deficiency. Thyroglobulin undergoes extracytosis to be stored in the lumen of the thyroid follicle. Storage is sufficient to last for about 2 months. Endocytosis of thyroglobulin, followed by phagolysosomal hydrolysis, starts the secretory process of the release of thyroid hormones into the circulation. Again, this is a TSH-dependent tightly controlled process. Non-secreted iodothyronines are metabolised to tyrosine and iodide. Apart from the thyroid hormones, small amounts of thyroglobulin reach the circulation. Daily thyroid hormone secretion of T4 and T3 has been estimated to be 100 μg and 10 μg, respectively [2]. We are not implying this is a fixed ratio though.

When released into the circulation, thyroid hormones are bound to *thyroid transport proteins* to facilitate their transport to the organs and prolong their half-life in the blood stream [18]. The plasma half-life of T4 is 5–7 days and that of T3 1–3 days, depending on various influences including thyroid function, with an extended half-life in hypothyroidism [19]. The fractions of circulating unbound *free T4* (*FT4*) and *free T3* (*FT3*) are very small, 0.03% for T4 and 0.3% for T3. Much larger fractions of the hormones are reversibly bound to proteins, namely *thyroxine-binding globulin* (*TBG*), *transthyretin* and *albumin*. Any changes in the concentrations of transport proteins, which occur due to genetic TBG deficiency, oestrogen effects in pregnancy and contraceptive pills - while affecting total T4 and T3 concentrations - do not alter the concentrations of the free hormones. The equilibrated release of T4 from TBG is a temperature-sensitive mechanism [20]. This provides a rapid homeostatic mechanism to adapt FT4 concentrations to metabolic needs in case of external temperature change, such as observed during hypothermia and torpor in small animals. Infections and fever will cause a rise in body temperature in humans to prompt an accelerated release of thyroxine, resulting in a reported 23% increase in the concentration of free thyroxine at 39.8 °C [20]. Reliable thyroid function testing for diagnostic purposes must rely on the measurement of the *free hormones*, *FT3* and *FT4* [21] (see Chap. 8).

3.2 Types of Thyroid Hormone Signalling

Thyroid hormones exert their respective effects via four distinct *signalling types* that differ in their biochemical actions, locations and hormone specificities [22]. The classical genomic effects are referred to as type 1 action, where thyroid hormones affect gene expression via the formation of complexes with nuclear thyroid hormone receptors (THRs) bound to DNA or RNA as monomer, dimer or heterodimer [23]. In type 2 action, hormone-receptor complexes act indirectly via adaptor proteins to control gene expression. Type 3 action denotes the binding of thyroid hormones to cytoplasmic receptors before the specific effects are mediated via second messengers (e.g. phosphoinositide 3-kinase-Ak strain transforming - mammalian target of rapamycin (PI3K/AKT/mTOR) or the Mitogen-Activated Protein Kinase (MAPK)). In type 4 action thyroid hormones bind to integrin receptors on the cell membrane. In the latter form of signalling, they do not have to cross the cell membrane [24]. The different receptors involved in thyroid hormone signalling are shown in Table 3.1. For clinical relevance in the treatment of patients, refer to Sect. 11.6.

Table 3.1 Receptors for thyroid hormones in the mammalian organism

Receptor	Location	Tissues
THRα1	Nucleus (types 1 and 2 action) and cytoplasm (type 3 action)	Predominantly heart, skeletal muscle
THRβ1	Nucleus (types 1 and 2 action) and cytoplasm (type 3 action)	Predominantly in central nervous system (CNS), pituitary, liver and adipose tissue
THRβ2	Nucleus (types 1 and 2 action) and cytoplasm (type 3 action)	Predominantly in CNS, pituitary, liver and adipose tissue
THRβ3	Nucleus (types 1 and 2 action) and cytoplasm (type 3 action)	Predominantly in CNS, pituitary, liver and adipose tissue
p43	Mitochondria (type 1 action)	All tissues with mitochondria
aVβ3	Cell membrane (type 4 action)	Several tissues. Relevant effects described for myocardial and tumour cells

Table 3.2 Thyroid hormone transporters

Transporter	Associated gene(s)	Transported hormones	Organ distribution
MCT8	*SLC16A2*	T4, T3, rT3, T2	Central nervous system, liver, kidney, heart, thyroid, eye, pituitary, placenta
MCT10	*SLC16A10*	T4, T3	Muscle tissue, oocytes, duodenum, pancreas
NTCP	*SLC10A1*	T4, T3, rT3, T2	Liver
OATP1A2	*SLCO1A2*	T4, T3, rT3, T2	Central nervous system, liver, kidney, heart, thyroid, eye, pituitary, placenta
OATP1B1	*SLCO1B1*	T4, T3	Liver
OATP1B3	*SLCO1B3*	T4, T3	Liver
OATP1C1	*SLCO1C1*	T4, T3, rT3	Central nervous system, cochlea, tests
OATP4A1	*SLCO4A1*	T4, T3, rT3	Placenta and multiple other tissues
OATP4C1	*SLCO4C1*	T3	Kidney and other tissues
LAT1	*SLC3A2 and SLC7A5* (heterodimer)	T4, T3, rT3, T2	Intestine and multiple other tissues including tumours
LAT2	*SLC3A2 and SLC7A8* (heterodimer)	T4, T3, rT3, T2	Intestine and multiple other tissues including tumours

MCT Monocarboxylate transporter, *NTCP* Sodium-taurocholate co-transporting peptide, *OATP* Organic anion transporting peptide, *LAT* Large neutral amino acid transporter

3.3 Transmembrane Transport and Intracellular Effects

Contrary to earlier assumptions, FT3 and FT4 in the circulation do not diffuse across plasma membranes but are transported by various specialised *transport proteins* [25] (Table 3.2). Intracellular trafficking then involves intracellular binding substrates (IBSs) of thyroid hormones (e.g., CRYM) [26]. Specialised transmembrane transport is also involved in the feedback control by thyroid hormones at the pituitary. This is particularly apparent in a rare syndrome of MCT8 deficiency, the *Allan-Herndon-Dudley syndrome* [27]. Transporters may be subject to regulation by T3 as has been shown in their hypothalamic expression in rodents [28].

However, transmembrane carriers are not the only way to transport thyroid hormones, especially FT3, from the plasma into the cell to exert genomic actions. Yet another pathway has only recently been discovered to specifically facilitate the transport of T3 in TRH neurons by *endosomal, non-degradative lysosomes* and retrograde transport to the nucleus [29]. T3 is thereby protected against degradation by the enzyme type 3 deiodinase, which is abundant in brain tissues. This novel pathway gives FT3 more weight than previously assumed in the balanced negative feedback by both thyroid hormones FT4 and FT3 on pituitary TSH secretion. Predictions of mathematical modelling agree with that notion [30] (Chap. 5).

T3 is the *biologically more active thyroid hormone*, compared to T4. The latter can be regarded both as a *precursor*, representing a *prohormone* to be activated in tissues via enzymatic T4 to T3 conversion (type 1 signalling) [31], and an active hormone binding to integrin receptors (type 4 signalling) [22]. Intracellular actions of thyroid hormones following their active transport across the plasma membrane are shown in Fig. 3.3 [23]. Various tissues differentially express three known types of *deiodinases*

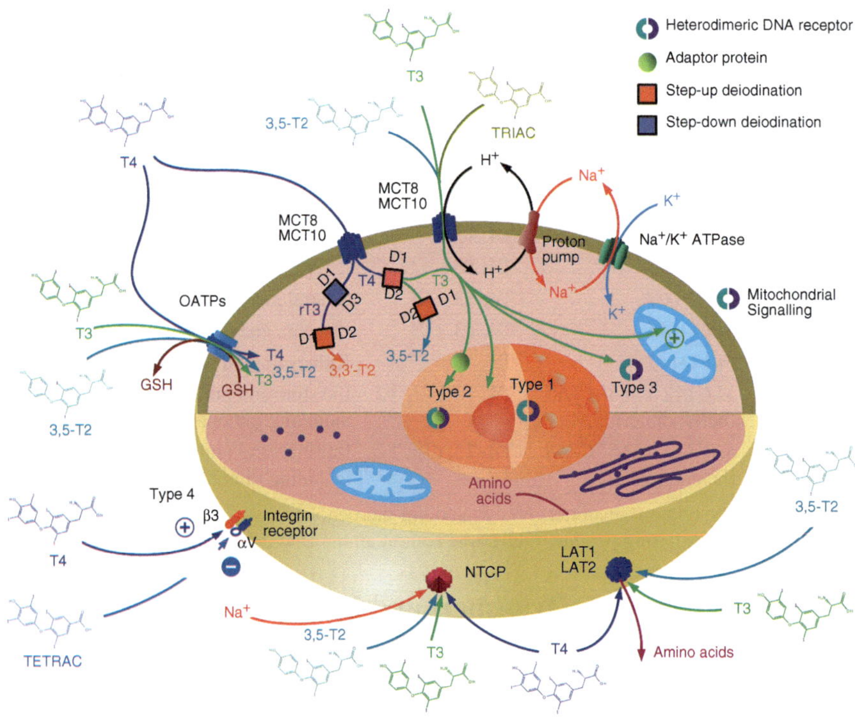

Fig. 3.3 Intracellular pathways and actions of thyroid hormones
Thyroid hormones are actively transported across the plasma membrane by various thyroid hormone transporters (Table 3.2). Deiodinases D1 and D2 are involved in converting T4 to the biologically more active T3 hormone. Deiodinase D1 and D3 further convert T3 to 3,5-T2. Deiodinase D3 inactivates T4 to rT3 and T3 to 3,3′-T2. T3 is transported in the cytosol to the nucleus and mitochondria, binding there to different thyroid hormone receptors (Table 3.3) and exerting different types of signalling. See text for details

[3, 32]. Type 1 deiodinase is mainly expressed in the thyroid, liver and kidneys and exhibits a relatively low affinity to T4. High-affinity type 2 deiodinase is primarily expressed by the central organs including the pituitary, brown fat tissue and also the thyroid. Expression of type 2 deiodinase allows for adaptive regulation of T3 availability to satisfy specific requirements at the level of each tissue. This becomes an important physiological consideration in the context of thyroid hormone replacement with levothyroxine, as will be discussed later. Type 3 deiodinase inactivates both T4 and T3. It is also the main source for the production of reverse T3 (rT3). The activities of deiodinases are regulated both by thyroid hormones themselves and partly by pituitary TSH. Hypothyroidism induces the expression of the type 2 enzyme to increase T4–T3 conversion, particularly in sensitive tissues such as the brain and pituitary. TSH is increased in primary hypothyroidism, resulting in the activation of a TSH-T3 shunt or TSH-T3 feed-forward control in TSH-sensitive tissues, including the thyroid itself [33–38]. Apart from TSH, the T4 to T3 conversion rate is influenced by many factors, such as fasting, obesity, severe disease, acute traumata, application of contrast agents and numerous drugs (propylthiouracil, propranolol, amiodarone, glucocorticoids). Large haemangiomas expressing type 3 deiodinase are a rare cause of hypothyroidism, particularly seen in children, termed consumptive hypothyroidism [39].

3.4 Mitochondria and T3 Actions

Thyroid hormones have long been recognised as important regulators of *body temperature* and *metabolic rate*. Their actions on *energy metabolism* involve the cellular apparatus where metabolic transformations take place, namely the mitochondria [5]. T3 regulation of mitochondriogenesis is likely to involve both nuclear and mitochondrial (p43) receptors [40–43]. Mechanisms of energy transduction, among others, activate the mitochondrial respiratory chain, which is organised in super-complexes and cristae. In isolated mitochondria, the so-called proton leak across the inner membrane is an important target of thyroid hormone to modulate oxygen consumption. In another pathway, subunit F1-ATPase of the mitochondrial complex synthesising ATP is encoded by genes whose expression is regulated by T3. T3 may also increase mitochondrial transcription factor (mt-TFA) to stimulate mt-DNA replication and expression. We refer the interested readers to dedicated reviews on novel insights and details on the complex mitochondrial regulatory system [40, 42]. However, much remains to be investigated on mechanisms of control and precisely how these actions are regulated.

We summarise that thyroid hormone actions increase oxygen consumption and heat production, and hypothyroidism exerts opposite effects. Hormonal regulation of mitochondrial activity influences both *ATP production* and *cell differentiation*, providing a link between metabolism and development. At the clinical level, impairments in energy metabolism and thermogenesis translate into typical symptoms of hypothyroidism such as cold intolerance and weight gain. Temperature differences to normal subjects may even persist in levothyroxine-treated patients [44].

Table 3.3 Types and characteristics of deiodinases

Property	Deiodinase type 1	Deiodinase type 2	Deiodinase type 3
Main sites of expression	Liver, kidney, thyroid	Pituitary, tanycytes, glial cells, thyroid, bone, brown adipose tissue, skeletal muscles	Brain, placenta, skin, haemangiomas
Cellular location	Plasma membrane	Endoplasmic reticulum	Plasma membrane
Main function	Activating role on T3–T4 conversion	Activating role on T3–T4 conversion Special role in thyroid hormone feedback Role in differentiation and development	Deactivating role on T4 (to reverse T3) and T3 (to T2)
Apparent dissociation constant of the enzyme (Km value)	10^{-6}–10^{-7} M	10^{-9} M	10^{-9} M
Regulatory influences	T4, T3, partly TSH, cAMP, cytokines	T4, T3, TSH, cAMP, FOXO3, bile acid, sympathetic nervous system, ubiquitination	HGH, glucocorticoids, TGF-ß, growth factors, HIF-1
Influence of thyroid function	Differentially regulated by T4 and T3 and in tissues, upregulated by T3, upregulated at the thyroid in hypothyroidism and hyperthyroidism, downregulated in liver in kidney and hypothyroidism	Upregulated in hypothyroidism and downregulated in hyperthyroidism	Downregulated in hypothyroidism and upregulated in hyperthyroidism
Pharmacological inhibitor	Propylthiouracil, Iopanoic acid	Iopanoic acid	Iopanoic acid

3.5 Deiodinases

Deiodinases are *selenoprotein enzymes* expressed by many—but not all—tissues, which remove one iodine molecule at a certain position from the tyrosine structure (monodeiodination) [3]. Their main task is either to activate or inactivate the hormone (Fig. 3.3). Three types of deiodinases are known which differ in their tempo-spatial expression, tissue distribution, intracellular location, biochemical properties and regulation [3, 31, 45–54] (Table 3.3). Important regulatory factors of deiodinase activity, among others, include the thyroid hormones themselves (T4, T3), calcium-phosphoinositol, cyclic adenosine monophosphate (cAMP), TSH, human chorionic gonadotropin (hCG), and TSH receptor-stimulating antibodies.

In the pituitary, organ-specific differential expression and regulation of type 2 deiodinase is particularly important [55]. This gland responds primarily to changes in the intracellular local T3 production (central T3). Central T3 is largely derived from circulating FT4 after the latter is locally converted into T3 through the action of type 2 deiodinase. Circulating FT3 originating from peripheral deiodinase activities is assumed to be less influential in this respect. However, a novel pathway of axonal T3 uptake by TRH neurons, dependent on the MCT8 transporter and endosomal/non-degradative lysosomes, has only recently been discovered [29]. This mechanism protects T3 during the transport to the cell nucleus against degradation by the strongly expressed type 3 deiodinase in the brain. Unlike peripheral deiodinase-expressing tissues, the pituitary increases the expression of type 2 deiodinase at high T4 concentrations in order to maintain T3 production and central T3 concentrations at a high level. The latter mechanism allows the pituitary to respond to increasing FT4 levels, thereby permitting appropriate TSH feedback. It involves a deiodinase type 2 ubiquitination-dependent pathway operating in a way unique to thyrotrophs [55].

The spatio-temporal separation and divergence between the central and peripheral T3 equilibrium has important implications for hypothalamic–pituitary–thyroid axis regulation (Chap. 5). For the clinical use of TSH as a diagnostic marker of thyroid function, this means that the TSH level is not merely reflective of peripheral thyroid function and therefore cannot be a reliable indicator of euthyroidism. Importantly, central T3 concentrations, as opposed to peripheral T3 concentrations, are enhanced by the activation of deiodinase type 2 [56], resulting in the suppression of TSH, and consequently reduction of thyroid hormone production and decrease of circulating FT4 and FT3 concentrations. This may, for instance, at least partly, explain why FT3 serum levels remain disproportionally low even when a supposedly normal TSH concentration has been achieved by means of LT4 replacement [56]. The resulting *disjoint* between TSH and FT3 that is observed in athyreotic patients on LT4 replacement has important clinical implications, namely that TSH concentrations within the accepted reference range may not necessarily and invariably signal optimum concentrations of peripherally active FT3 (see Chap. 2). Consequently, the thyroid status and dose adequacy of LT4 substitution cannot readily be defined in these conditions merely on the basis of the TSH level. This will be an important issue of discussion in the section on the treatment of hypothyroidism.

References

1. Mantzouratou P, Lavecchia AM, Xinaris C. Thyroid hormone signaling in human evolution and disease: a novel hypothesis. J Clin Med. 2021;11:43. https://doi.org/10.3390/jcm11010043.
2. Bianco AC, Dumitrescu A, Gereben B, Ribeiro MO, Fonseca TL, Fernandes GW, Bocco BMLC. Paradigms of dynamic control of thyroid hormone signaling. Endocr Rev. 2019;40:1000–47. https://doi.org/10.1210/er.2018-00275.

3. Gereben B, Zavacki AM, Ribich S, Kim BW, Huang SA, Simonides WS, Zeöld A, Bianco AC. Cellular and molecular basis of deiodinase-regulated thyroid hormone signaling. Endocr Rev. 2008;29:898–938. https://doi.org/10.1210/er.2008-0019.
4. Hoermann R, Midgley JEM, Larisch R, Dietrich JW. Homeostatic control of the thyroid-pituitary axis: perspectives for diagnosis and treatment. Front Endocrinol (Lausanne). 2015;6:177. https://doi.org/10.3389/fendo.2015.00177.
5. Silvestri E, Schiavo L, Lombardi A, Goglia F. Thyroid hormones as molecular determinants of thermogenesis. Acta Physiol Scand. 2005;184:265–83. https://doi.org/10.1111/j.1365-201X.2005.01463.x.
6. Zucchi R, Chiellini G, Scanlan TS, Grandy DK. Trace amine-associated receptors and their ligands. Br J Pharmacol. 2006;149:967–78. https://doi.org/10.1038/sj.bjp.0706948.
7. Piehl S, Hoefig CS, Scanlan TS, Köhrle J. Thyronamines—past, present, and future. Endocr Rev. 2011;32:64–80. https://doi.org/10.1210/er.2009-0040.
8. Führer D, Brix K, Biebermann H. Thyroid hormone action beyond classical concepts. The priority programme "thyroid trans act" (spp 1629) of the German research foundation. Dtsch Med Wochenschr. 2014;139:492–6. https://doi.org/10.1055/s-0034-1369822.
9. Dietrich JW, Müller P, Schiedat F, Schlömicher M, Strauch J, Chatzitomaris A, Klein HH, Mügge A, Köhrle J, Rijntjes E, Lehmphul I. Nonthyroidal illness syndrome in cardiac illness involves elevated concentrations of 3,5-diiodothyronine and correlates with atrial remodeling. Eur Thyroid J. 2015;4:129–37. https://doi.org/10.1159/000381543.
10. Hoefig CS, Zucchi R, Köhrle J. Thyronamines and derivatives: physiological relevance, pharmacological actions, and future research directions. Thyroid. 2016;26:1656–73. https://doi.org/10.1089/thy.2016.0178.
11. Köhrle J, Biebermann H. 3-iodothyronamine-a thyroid hormone metabolite with distinct target profiles and mode of action. Endocr Rev. 2019;40:602–30. https://doi.org/10.1210/er.2018-00182.
12. Rosenfeld L. Discovery and early uses of iodine. J Chem Educ. 2000;77:984. https://doi.org/10.1021/ed077p984.
13. Zimmermann MB. Iodine deficiency. Endocr Rev. 2009;30:376–408. https://doi.org/10.1210/er.2009-0011.
14. Dai G, Levy O, Carrasco N. Cloning and characterization of the thyroid iodide transporter. Nature. 1996;379:458–60. https://doi.org/10.1038/379458a0.
15. Spitzweg C, Morris JC. The sodium iodide symporter: its pathophysiological and therapeutic implications. Clin Endocrinol. 2002;57:559–74.
16. Jing L, Zhang Q. Intrathyroidal feedforward and feedback network regulating thyroid hormone synthesis and secretion. Front Endocrinol (Lausanne). 2022;13:992883. https://doi.org/10.3389/fendo.2022.992883.
17. Citterio CE, Targovnik HM, Arvan P. The role of thyroglobulin in thyroid hormonogenesis. Nat Rev Endocrinol. 2019;15:323–38. https://doi.org/10.1038/s41574-019-0184-8.
18. Schussler GC. The thyroxine-binding proteins. Thyroid. 2000;10:141–9. https://doi.org/10.1089/thy.2000.10.141.
19. Colucci P, Yue CS, Ducharme M, Benvenga S. A review of the pharmacokinetics of levothyroxine for the treatment of hypothyroidism. Eur Endocrinol. 2013;9:40–7. https://doi.org/10.17925/EE.2013.09.01.40.
20. Qi X, Chan WL, Read RJ, Zhou A, Carrell RW. Temperature-responsive release of thyroxine and its environmental adaptation in Australians. Proc Biol Sci. 2014;281:20132747. https://doi.org/10.1098/rspb.2013.2747.
21. Midgley JEM. Direct and indirect free thyroxine assay methods: theory and practice. Clin Chem. 2001;47:1353–63.
22. Flamant F, Cheng SY, Hollenberg AN, Moeller LC, Samarut J, Wondisford FE, Yen PM, Refetoff S. Thyroid hormone signaling pathways: time for a more precise nomenclature. Endocrinology. 2017;158:2052–7. https://doi.org/10.1210/en.2017-00250.

23. Cheng S-Y, Leonard JL, Davis PJ. Molecular aspects of thyroid hormone actions. Endocr Rev. 2010;31:139–70. https://doi.org/10.1210/er.2009-0007.
24. Hercbergs A. Clinical implications and impact of discovery of the thyroid hormone receptor on integrin αvβ3—a review. Front Endocrinol (Lausanne). 2019;10:565. https://doi.org/10.3389/fendo.2019.00565.
25. Groeneweg S, Van Geest FS, Peeters RP, Heuer H, Visser WE. Thyroid hormone transporters. Endocr Rev. 2020;41:bnz008. https://doi.org/10.1210/endrev/bnz008.
26. Takeshige K, Sekido T, Kitahara J-I, Ohkubo Y, Hiwatashi D, Ishii H, Nishio S-I, Takeda T, Komatsu M, Suzuki S. Cytosolic T3-binding protein modulates dynamic alteration of T3-mediated gene expression in cells. Endocr J. 2014;61:561–70. https://doi.org/10.1507/endocrj.ej13-0418.
27. Schwartz CE, May MM, Carpenter NJ, Rogers RC, Martin J, Bialer MG, Ward J, Sanabria J, Marsa S, Lewis JA. Allan-Herndon-Dudley syndrome and the monocarboxylate transporter 8 (mct8) gene. Am J Hum Genet. 2005;77:41–53. https://doi.org/10.1086/431313.
28. Herwig A, Campbell G, Mayer C-D, Boelen A, Anderson RA, Ross AW, Mercer JG, Barrett P. A thyroid hormone challenge in hypothyroid rats identifies T3 regulated genes in the hypothalamus and in models with altered energy balance and glucose homeostasis. Thyroid. 2014;24:1575–93. https://doi.org/10.1089/thy.2014.0169.
29. Salas-Lucia F, Fekete C, Sinkó R, Egri P, Rada K, Ruska Y, Gereben B, Bianco AC. Axonal T3 uptake and transport can trigger thyroid hormone signaling in the brain. elife. 2023;12:e82683. https://doi.org/10.7554/eLife.82683.
30. Hoermann R, Pekker M, Midgley JEM, Larisch R, Dietrich JW. Principles of endocrine regulation: reconciling tensions between robustness in performance and adaptation to change. Front Endocrinol (Lausanne). 2022;13:825107. https://doi.org/10.3389/fendo.2022.825107.
31. Bianco AC, Salvatore D, Gereben B, Berry MJ, Larsen PR. Biochemistry, cellular and molecular biology, and physiological roles of the iodothyronine selenodeiodinases. Endocr Rev. 2002;23:38–89. https://doi.org/10.1210/edrv.23.1.0455.
32. Larsen PR, Zavacki AM. The role of the iodothyronine deiodinases in the physiology and pathophysiology of thyroid hormone action. Eur Thyroid J. 2012;1:232–42. https://doi.org/10.1159/000343922.
33. Ishii H, Inada M, Tanaka K, Mashio Y, Naito K, Nishikawa M, Matsuzuka F, Kuma K, Imura H. Induction of outer and inner ring monodeiodinases in human thyroid gland by thyrotropin. J Clin Endocrinol Metab. 1983;57:500–5. https://doi.org/10.1210/jcem-57-3-500.
34. Toyoda N, Nishikawa M, Mori Y, Gondou A, Ogawa Y, Yonemoto T, Yoshimura M, Masaki H, Inada M. Thyrotropin and triiodothyronine regulate iodothyronine 5′-deiodinase messenger ribonucleic acid levels in frtl-5 rat thyroid cells. Endocrinology. 1992;131:389–94. https://doi.org/10.1210/endo.131.1.1319323.
35. Beech SG, Walker SW, Arthur JR, Lee D, Beckett GJ. Differential control of type-i iodothyronine deiodinase expression by the activation of the cyclic amp and phosphoinositol signaling pathways in cultured human thyrocytes. J Mol Endocrinol. 1995;14:171–7. https://doi.org/10.1677/jme.0.0140171.
36. Koenig RJ. Regulation of type 1 iodothyronine deiodinase in health and disease. Thyroid. 2005;15:835–40. https://doi.org/10.1089/thy.2005.15.835.
37. Hoermann R, Midgley JEM, Larisch R, Dietrich JW. Relational stability in the expression of normality, variation, and control of thyroid function. Front Endocrinol (Lausanne). 2016;7:142. https://doi.org/10.3389/fendo.2016.00142.
38. Berberich J, Dietrich JW, Hoermann R, Müller MA. Mathematical modeling of the pituitary-thyroid feedback loop: role of a TSH-t3-shunt and sensitivity analysis. Front Endocrinol (Lausanne). 2018;9:91. https://doi.org/10.3389/fendo.2018.00091.
39. Luongo C, Trivisano L, Alfano F, Salvatore D. Type 3 deiodinase and consumptive hypothyroidism: a common mechanism for a rare disease. Front Endocrinol (Lausanne). 2013;4:115. https://doi.org/10.3389/fendo.2013.00115.

40. Iwen KA, Oelkrug R, Brabant G. Effects of thyroid hormones on thermogenesis and energy partitioning. J Mol Endocrinol. 2018;60:R157–70. https://doi.org/10.1530/jme-17-0319.
41. Goglia F, Moreno M, Lanni A. Action of thyroid hormones at the cellular level: the mitochondrial target. FEBS Lett. 1999;452:115–20. https://doi.org/10.1016/S0014-5793(99)00642-0.
42. Wrutniak-Cabello C, Casas F, Cabello G. Thyroid hormone action in mitochondria. J Mol Endocrinol. 2001;26:67–77. https://doi.org/10.1677/jme.0.0260067.
43. Cioffi F, Giacco A, Goglia F, Silvestri E. Bioenergetic aspects of mitochondrial actions of thyroid hormones. Cells. 2022;11:997. https://doi.org/10.3390/cells11060997.
44. Romero-Ibarguengoitia ME, Garza-Silva A, Rivera-Cavazos A, Morales-Rodriguez DP, González-Peña OI, Barco-Flores IA, Manilla-Muñoz E, Villarreal-Leal E, González-Cantú A. Temperature differences between controlled primary hypothyroidism and healthy patients: an exploratory study. J Endocr Soc. 2024;8:bvad175. https://doi.org/10.1210/jendso/bvad175.
45. Dentice M, Salvatore D. Local impact of thyroid hormone inactivation: deiodinases: the balance of thyroid hormone. J Endocrinol. 2011;209:273–82. https://doi.org/10.1530/JOE-11-0002.
46. Marsili A, Zavacki AM, Harney JW, Larsen PR. Physiological role and regulation of iodothyronine deiodinases: a 2011 update. J Endocrinol Investig. 2011;34:395–407. https://doi.org/10.1007/BF03347465.
47. Araujo RL, Carvalho DP. Bioenergetic impact of tissue-specific regulation of iodothyronine deiodinases during nutritional imbalance. J Bioenerg Biomembr. 2011;43:59–65. https://doi.org/10.1007/s10863-011-9327-x.
48. Maia AL, Goemann IM, Meyer ELS, Wajner SM. Type 1 iodothyronine deiodinase in human physiology and disease: deiodinases: the balance of thyroid hormone. J Endocrinol. 2011;209:283–97. https://doi.org/10.1530/JOE-10-0481.
49. Williams GR, Bassett JHD. Local control of thyroid hormone action: role of type 2 deiodinase: deiodinases: the balance of thyroid hormone. J Endocrinol. 2011;209:261–72. https://doi.org/10.1530/JOE-10-0448.
50. Gereben B, Mcaninch EA, Ribeiro MO, Bianco AC. Scope and limitations of iodothyronine deiodinases in hypothyroidism. Nat Rev Endocrinol. 2015;11:642–52. https://doi.org/10.1038/nrendo.2015.155.
51. Schweizer U, Steegborn C. New insights into the structure and mechanism of iodothyronine deiodinases. J Mol Endocrinol. 2015;55:R37–52. https://doi.org/10.1530/JME-15-0156.
52. Luongo C, Dentice M, Salvatore D. Deiodinases and their intricate role in thyroid hormone homeostasis. Nat Rev Endocrinol. 2019;15:479–88. https://doi.org/10.1038/s41574-019-0218-2.
53. Russo SC, Salas-Lucia F, Bianco AC. Deiodinases and the metabolic code for thyroid hormone action. Endocrinology. 2021;162:bqab059. https://doi.org/10.1210/endocr/bqab059/6171212.
54. Deng Y, Han Y, Gao S, Dong W, Yu Y. The physiological functions and polymorphisms of type ii deiodinase. Endocrinol Metab (Seoul). 2023;38:190–202. https://doi.org/10.3803/EnM.2022.1599.
55. Werneck De Castro JP, Fonseca TL, Ueta CB, Mcaninch EA, Abdalla SM, Wittmann G, Lechan RM, Gereben B, Bianco AC. Differences in hypothalamic type 2 deiodinase ubiquitination explain localized sensitivity to thyroxine. J Clin Invest. 2015;125:769–81. https://doi.org/10.1172/JCI77588.
56. Hoermann R, Midgley JEM, Larisch R, Dietrich JW. Is pituitary TSH an adequate measure of thyroid hormone-controlled homoeostasis during thyroxine treatment. Eur J Endocrinol. 2013;168:271–80. https://doi.org/10.1530/EJE-12-0819.

Chapter 4
Introduction to Mathematical Modelling

Mark J. Pekker-Friedman

4.1 What Are Mathematical Models

Mathematical models determine how the system changes from one state to the next and describe the interdependence of the variables (or factors) involved. In contrast, statistical analyses characterise numerical data and attempt at estimating probabilistic future behaviour of a system based on its past behaviour. Mathematical models are generally exact and given by equations, whereas statistical models are generally given by data and the probability of the dataset matching the statistical assumptions. Some goals may be shared between the two approaches, but the key difference between mathematical models and statistical models lies in their underlying assumptions and objectives. Mathematical models are based on established principles, laws, and theories of the physical world. They aim to describe and predict the behaviour of a system using mathematical equations and relationships. These models typically involve variables, parameters, and deterministic functions that capture the underlying mechanics and dynamics of the system. The goal of a mathematical model is to provide a comprehensive, theoretically grounded representation of the system.

On the other hand, statistical models are primarily data-driven. They are used to analyse and make inferences from observed data, often with the aim of identifying patterns, trends, and relationships. Statistical models rely on probability distributions, hypothesis testing, and estimation techniques to quantify the uncertainty and variability inherent in the data. The goal of a statistical model is to summarise the data, test hypotheses, and make predictions based on the observed data and statistical assumptions.

M. J. Pekker-Friedman (✉)
Mathematical Sciences Department, University of Alabama, Huntsville, AL, USA
e-mail: mark.pekker@uah.edu

R. Hoermann, J. W. Dietrich (eds.), *Hypothyroidism*,
https://doi.org/10.1007/978-981-96-3682-2_4

In summary, mathematical models focus on the underlying mechanisms and deterministic relationships, while statistical models focus on the patterns, trends, and probabilistic relationships within the data. Both approaches have their own strengths and applications, and they are often used in complementary ways to understand and analyse complex systems, as is the case in chapters of the book dedicated to the regulation of the thyroid system.

4.2 Mathematical Modelling in Individualised Medicine

Personalised medicine aims to provide tailor-made prevention and treatment strategies for defined groups of individuals. Individualised medicine represents a further individualisation of personalised medicine. While the latter is aimed at a specific group of patients, individualised medicine deals with the individual circumstances of a single person. Particularly in individualised medicine, mathematical models can help researchers uncover and understand mechanisms of health and disease beyond statistical association. They can also uncover emergent phenomena that are otherwise obscured in highly complex networks. Thereby, predictive mathematical models can lead to new refined treatment protocols and drugs and improve disease prevention and diagnosis.

4.2.1 Mathematical Modelling of the Endocrine System

Mechanistic mathematical models based on differential equations are useful to reflect our present-level understanding of the functional interactions that determine the overall behaviour of the system under investigation (in our case, the endocrine system or more specifically thyroid system) [1]. By casting our knowledge of physiology in the framework of dynamical systems, we enable both qualitative and precise quantitative predictions to be made and to be compared against results from suitably chosen experiments. Such mathematical models often allow us to probe a system in much greater detail than is possible in experimental studies. They can therefore help establish the cause and causal relationships behind a particular clinical observation. When integrated into a clinical programme, mathematical models and experiments are highly synergistic, in that the existence of one greatly enhances the value of the other. Models not only depend on experiments for specification and refinement of parameter values, but they also illuminate experimental observations, allow for differentiation between competing scientific hypotheses and alternative mechanisms, and help aid in experimental design. Analysing models rigorously, through sensitivity and/or numerical bifurcation analyses [2], or simple simulations of what-if scenarios also allows for identification of crucial gaps in our knowledge and therefore help motivate the design of targeted experiments. In summary, mathematical modelling of complex systems, such as the endocrine system and in particular the hypothalamic–pituitary–thyroid axis regulation is an essential step towards increasing our knowledge of the inner working and underlying mechanisms of a highly complex network of hormonal interactions.

Endocrine systems are *control systems*, where control signals are hormones that are distributed between endocrine glands via circulation. They can typically be described by the present state and an equation of motion that depends on the current state of the system. *Mathematical modelling* is a process for formulating a set of equations to simultaneously represent a system's structure and behaviour. In most cases, the equations of the mathematical model are non-linear *ordinary differential equations* (ODEs). Such models offer insights into the mechanisms and signal transduction pathways and provide the bedrock for hypothesis-generating research. This has been exemplified in the thyroid system [1]. Furthermore, the parameters of the model may conveniently serve as biomarkers of specific biological mechanisms, or of pathophysiological states. Qualitative behaviours of autonomous ODE systems may include convergence to *equilibrium points* or *steady states*, which are states at which all variables remain constant.

These aspects will be expanded on in more detail and discussed in clinical context in Chap. 5 dedicated to Hypothalamic–Pituitary–Thyroid Regulation.

4.3 Operationalisation of Homeostasis and Allostasis

It may be helpful to provide *operational definitions* for some concepts and terms that are important for our understanding of mathematical models of the hypothalamic–pituitary–thyroid regulation, as presented in Chap. 5.

4.3.1 Homeostasis

Homeostasis is concerned with regulatory mechanisms, present in biological systems, where *some specific variable is kept close to a set value* as some external disturbance affects the system [3, 4]. In all these cases there are homeostatic regions where the variable is relatively insensitive to external stimulus, flanked by regions where it is sensitive.

Allostasis, on the other hand, is primarily concerned with the same regulatory mechanisms in relation to a *biological system as a whole* including its evolution or adaptive change.

Mathematically, the notion of homeostasis can be formalised in terms of an *input-output function* that maps the parameter representing the external disturbance to the output variable that must be kept within a fairly narrow range [3, 4]. The derivative of the input-output function is zero at an isolated point. An *input-output network* is a network with two distinguished nodes *input* and *output*, and the dynamics of the network determines the corresponding input-output function of the system.

In this mathematical framework, one considers a system of parametrised differential equations:

$$\frac{dX}{dt} = F(X,\alpha), \tag{4.1}$$

with the corresponding equilibrium system

$$F(X,\alpha) = 0. \tag{4.2}$$

Here X is a *state vector variable,* and α is an *input parameter* representing the external input to the system.

Definition 4.1 Input-output function $X(\alpha)$ is defined as follows. Suppose that (X_0, α_0) is a linearly stable equilibrium of (Eq. 4.1), i.e. $F(X_0, \alpha_0) = 0$, and all eigenvalues λ of the Jacobian matrix $J = (DF)(X_0, \alpha_0)$ have $\text{Re}\lambda < 0$. And let $X(\alpha)$ be family of linearly stable equilibria such that $X(\alpha_0) = X_0$ and $F(X(\alpha), \alpha) \equiv 0$.

As an example of system (Eq. 4.2), we consider some 4-dim systems in [1] and [5].

In this case, X = ([TRH], [TSH], [FT4], [FT3]) is a (vector) state variable. And we consider homeostasis of the fourth component [FT3] of X. This means that FT3 concentration changes by a relatively small amount when the parameter, say, α = k32, the FT4 production rate constant varies by a much larger amount, and another internal variable, say, FT4 or TSH, also varies by a much larger amount.

For convenience of presentation, we will use from now on the notation

$$X = (Y,z), Y = (y_1,y_2,y_3) = ([\text{TRH}],[\text{TSH}],[\text{FT4}]), z = [\text{FT3}]$$

and rewrite Eq. (4.2) as

$$F(Y,z,\alpha) = 0. \tag{4.3}$$

In this situation, we say that the system (Eq. 4.3) exhibits *homeostasis* if, under variation of the input parameter α, the input-output function $z(\alpha)$ remains approximately constant over the interval of external stimuli.

Homeostasis and allostasis can be operationalised in the language of dynamical systems, numerical bifurcation analysis, and numerical linear algebra.

Definition 4.2 Homeostasis

- α_0 is a *Homeostasis Point* if $z'(\alpha_0) = 0$, and $z(\alpha_0)$ is a *Homeostatic State*
- $z(\alpha)$ exhibits *Perfect Homeostasis* on a *Homeostatic Interval* (or *Region*) (α_-, α_+), if $z'(\alpha) = 0$ for all $\alpha \in (\alpha_-, \alpha_+)$
- $z(\alpha)$ exhibits *δ-Homeostasis* relative to a *Set Point* $\alpha_0 \in (\alpha_-, \alpha_+)$ if, for fixed δ, for all α, $|z(\alpha) - z(\alpha_0)| \leq \delta$, $\alpha \in (\alpha_-, \alpha_+)$, a *$\delta$-Homeostatic Interval.*

In other words, a set point is the value about which homeostasis is approximately constant.

Remark A *Homeostasis Point* and a *Homeostatic State* can be detected and accurately located by numerical continuation and bifurcation software, such as [2].

4.3.2 Escape from Homeostasis

Escape from Homeostasis occurs when an eigenvalue λ of the Jacobian matrix J crosses the imaginary axis or satisfies Re $\lambda > 0$, and/or α gets out of the range (α_-, α_+).

Explanation. In our model, see Definition 4.1, the input parameter α represents the challenges due to external disturbances affecting a biological system. The regulatory mechanisms in such a system typically work only when these challenges are within a finite range. Outside that range, the mechanisms become ineffective, and the variables that the mechanisms are supposed to control change rapidly, a phenomenon that Nijhout et al. [6] call "escape from homeostasis." Clinically, *Escape from Homeostasis* may lead to an onset of symptoms of a disease.

4.3.3 Robustness of a Homeostatic State

Waddington postulated that mechanisms have evolved that stabilise the phenotype against both genetic and environmental perturbation [7]. He called this "canalisation" and contrasted that with developmental "flexibility" in which a phenotype changes, adaptively, with a change in environment [7]. Today we call these phenomena *robustness* and *adaptive plasticity*, respectively.

Robustness is an ability to resist otherwise deleterious genetic or environmental variation [8]. Robustness is an observed property of a system but does not imply a particular mechanism. Typical mechanisms of Robustness are feedback inhibition and feed-forward excitation type.

We define two measures of Robustness:

- Robustness as an amount of *dynamical compensation* of a *homeostatic state* is measured by the size of the real part $|\mathrm{Re}\lambda|$ of the eigenvalue $\lambda(\mathrm{Re}\lambda < 0)$ of the Jacobian matrix closest to the imaginary axis. The larger $|\mathrm{Re}\lambda|$, the higher is the robustness of the homeostatic state J and if $\mathrm{Re}\lambda = 0$, there is no robustness.

Explanation. The larger the $|\mathrm{Re}\lambda|$, the faster the *homeostatic state* is restored after the deleterious variation is removed.

- Robustness as an amount of *detrimental variation* of the mechanism of a *homeostatic state* measured by the magnitude of the smallest singular value $\sigma_{\min}$ (can be computed for instance in MATLAB, Mathworks Inc., Natick, MA, USA) of the Jacobian matrix $J = (\mathrm{DF})(X_0, \alpha_0)$.

Explanation. $\sigma_{\min}$ is the size (in 2-matrix norm) of the smallest perturbation ΔJ of the matrix J that can make $J + \Delta J$ singular and thus result in a breakdown of the Homeostatic State $z(\alpha_0)$.

Combining the above, we can define

$$\text{Robustness} = \left(\alpha_0, \alpha_+ - \alpha_-, |\text{Re}\lambda|, \sigma_{\min}\right), \tag{4.4}$$

where $\alpha_+ - \alpha_-$ is the length of δ-Homeostatic Interval. The larger each component of Robustness is, the higher Robustness is. The closer α_0 is to the middle of the interval (α_-, α_+), the higher Robustness is. We also define

$$\text{Type1Resilience} \equiv \text{Robustness}.$$

4.3.4 *Allostasis*

We will next extend our operationalisation of Homeostasis to include Allostasis. According to Bettinger and Friston [9], "[i]t is natural to regard both allostatic-load and allostatic-repair as implicit features of physiological homeostasis…".

- *Allostatic Process* is the process of an emergence and evolution of a system

$$\frac{dX_p}{dt} = F_p\left(X_p, a_p\right), \tag{4.5}$$

$$F_p\left(X_p, a_p\right) = 0 \tag{4.6}$$

which is a perturbation of the system (Eqs. 4.1 and 4.2) due to a stressor or triggering causes.

[Allostatic process → Allostatic Point and Allostatic state].

Let (X_{p0}, α_{p0}) be a linearly stable equilibrium of (Eq. 4.5), i.e. a solution of (Eq. 4.6). Then α_{p0} is an *Allostatic Point* if $z'(\alpha_{p0}) = 0$, and $z(\alpha_{p0})$ is the corresponding *Allostatic State.*

Explanation. Stressor or triggering causes are any characterisable factor or quantifiable characteristics of the system capable of registering within a perceptual space (in experience) or instrumentation.

Allostatic State accounts for quantifiable physiological and biochemical etc. effects of Allostatic Process; impairing or adaptive [Allostatic process → Allostatic load].

- *Allostatic Load* is measured by the difference $\sigma_{\min} - \sigma_{p,\min}$, where $\sigma_{\min}$ is defined above and $\sigma_{p,\min}$, defined analogously, is the magnitude of the smallest singular value $\sigma_{p,\min}$ of the Jacobian matrix $J_p = (DF_p)(X_{p0}, \alpha_{p0})$.

Explanation. A quantitative measure of the change of the total system, due to an allostatic process, resulting or not in a change of the homeostatic state.

- *Allostatic Overload.* (X_{p0}, α_{p0}) is no longer a linearly stable equilibrium, i.e. a bifurcation and the corresponding Escape from or Breakdown of Homeostasis have occurred.

Explanation. When aberrant allostatic load becomes pathological, crossing a tacit threshold from impairing to pathological, an upper bound of *allostatic impairment,* thereby leading to pathophysiological conditions.

4.3.5 Two Types of Allostatic Processes

- *Type 1 Allostatic Process* [9]. Repeated stressors produce an increasing allostatic load (in our example resulting in changes in FT4 and TSH levels) that can ultimately lead to a disease state and to "the cumulative cost to the body of allostasis, with allostatic overload being a state in which serious pathophysiology can occur" [10], in our example, escape from FT3 homeostasis. Monitoring the Allostatic Process by the Robustness parameters, see Eq. (4.4), would assist the clinician to uncover this process at an early stage when it may still be easy to reverse it before any symptoms appearing.
- *Type 2 Allostatic Process.* Now consider a scenario where it is difficult or impossible to arrest or reverse the allostatic process (in our example, changes in FT4 and TSH levels). In Hoermann et al. [1], an adaptation of the physiological circuits responsible for the hypothalamic–pituitary–thyroid regulation was identified which supports the preservation of FT3 homeostasis in the above case.
- *Type 2 Resilience.* The regulatory circuits are adapted to preserve FT3 homeostasis.

To summarise, combined types 1 and 2 resiliencies constitute an optimum resilience in stressful situations.

4.3.6 Choosing Between Homeostasis and Allostasis

While a formal distinction between the concepts of homeostasis and allostasis is useful, we propose a unified approach in the situational execution and expression of critical design principles at the system level in thyroid health and disease [1]. The thyroid system serves a dual goal in humans in providing a stable internal environment for the many energy- and temperature-dependent enzymatic reactions of the body and in synchronising transitions between their energetic and metabolic states in response to changing internal or external conditions [11]. This poses specific challenges to the thyroid system and its regulation in the event of a thyroid disease, in non-thyroidal disease, and in treated patients, particularly in those individuals with persistent hypothyroid symptoms, to be discussed in other chapters [12, 13].

References

1. Hoermann R, Pekker M, Midgley JEM, Larisch R, Dietrich JW. Principles of endocrine regulation: reconciling tensions between robustness in performance and adaptation to change. Front Endocrinol (Lausanne). 2022;13:825107. https://doi.org/10.3389/fendo.2022.825107.
2. Bindel D, Friedman M, Govaerts W, Hughes J, Kuznetsov Y. Numerical computation of bifurcations in large equilibrium systems in MATLAB. J Comput Appl Math. 2014;261:232–48. https://doi.org/10.1016/j.cam.2013.10.034.
3. Golubitsky M, Stewart I. Homeostasis, singularities, and networks. J Math Biol. 2017;74:387–407. https://doi.org/10.1007/s00285-016-1024-2.
4. Antoneli F, Golubitsky M, Jin J, Stewart I. Homeostasis in input-output networks: structure, classification and applications. arXiv. 2024:2405.03861v1.
5. Hoermann R, Pekker MJ, Midgley JEM, Dietrich JW. The role of supporting and disruptive mechanisms of FT3 homeostasis in regulating the hypothalamic-pituitary-thyroid axis. Ther Adv Endocrinol Metab. 2023;14:20420188231158163. https://doi.org/10.1177/20420188231158163.
6. Nijhout HF, Best J, Reed MC. Escape from homeostasis. Math Biosci. 2014;257:104–10. https://doi.org/10.1016/j.mbs.2014.08.015.
7. Waddington CH. The strategy of the genes: a discussion of some aspects of theoretical biology. London: Allen & Unwin; 1957.
8. Nijhout HF, Sadre-Marandi F, Best J, Reed MC. Systems biology of phenotypic robustness and plasticity. Integr Comp Biol. 2017;57:171–84. https://doi.org/10.1093/icb/icx076.
9. Bettinger JS, Friston KJ. Conceptual foundations of physiological regulation incorporating the free energy principle and self-organized criticality. Neurosci Biobehav Rev. 2023;155:105459. https://doi.org/10.1016/j.neubiorev.2023.105459.
10. Mcewen BS, Wingfield JC. The concept of allostasis in biology and biomedicine. Horm Behav. 2003;43:2–15.
11. Zwahlen J, Gairin E, Vianello S, Mercader M, Roux N, Laudet V. The ecological function of thyroid hormones. Philos Trans R Soc Lond Ser B Biol Sci. 2024;379:20220511. https://doi.org/10.1098/rstb.2022.0511.
12. Hoermann R, Midgley JEM, Larisch R, Dietrich JW. Homeostatic control of the thyroid-pituitary axis: perspectives for diagnosis and treatment. Front Endocrinol (Lausanne). 2015;6:177. https://doi.org/10.3389/fendo.2015.00177.
13. Chatzitomaris A, Hoermann R, Midgley JEM, Hering S, Urban A, Dietrich B, Abood A, Klein HH, Dietrich JW. Thyroid allostasis-adaptive responses of thyrotropic feedback control to conditions of strain, stress, and developmental programming. Front Endocrinol (Lausanne). 2017;8:163. https://doi.org/10.3389/fendo.2017.00163.

Chapter 5
Hypothalamic–Pituitary–Thyroid Regulation

Rudolf Hoermann and Johannes W. Dietrich

The ability of the organism to flexibly preserve *homeostatic equilibria* in response to internal or environmental challenges is a sign of its healthy state. Thyroid hormones target a broad spectrum of metabolic effects. This requires them to be tightly controlled, as are their energetic and metabolic targets. The involvement of pituitary thyrotropin (TSH) in thyroid hormone control has long been recognised [1]. As a result, the measurement of TSH has been exploited for the diagnosis of thyroid disorders, particularly after highly sensitive TSH assays became available in the 1980s [2–4]. Despite being at best an indirect indicator of thyroid hormone homeostasis, TSH measurement has become a corner stone of contemporary thyroid function testing [5, 6].

In recent years, our knowledge of the mechanisms involved in the regulation of thyroid hormones has greatly evolved. The underlying system is far more complex than previously thought (Fig. 5.1). This requires a revision of long-held simplistic concepts and promotes a multifactorial concept of the feedback control between the

---

R. Hoermann (✉)
Yandina, QLD, Australia

Department of General Internal Medicine, Gastroenterology and Endocrinology, [Retired] Klinikum Lüdenscheid, Lüdenscheid, Germany
e-mail: rudolf.hoermann@gmail.com

J. W. Dietrich
Diabetes, Endocrinology and Metabolism Section, Department of Medicine, St. Josef-Hospital, Ruhr University Hospitals, Bochum, Germany

Centre for Diabetes Technology (ZDT), Catholic Hospitals Bochum, Bochum, Germany

Centre for Rare Endocrine Diseases (ZSEK), Ruhr Center for Rare Diseases (CeSER), Ruhr University of Bochum and Witten/Herdecke University, Bochum, Germany

Centre for Thyroid Medicine (ZSM), Ruhr University of Bochum, Bochum, Germany
e-mail: johannes.dietrich@ruhr-uni-bochum.de

R. Hoermann, J. W. Dietrich (eds.), *Hypothyroidism*,
https://doi.org/10.1007/978-981-96-3682-2_5

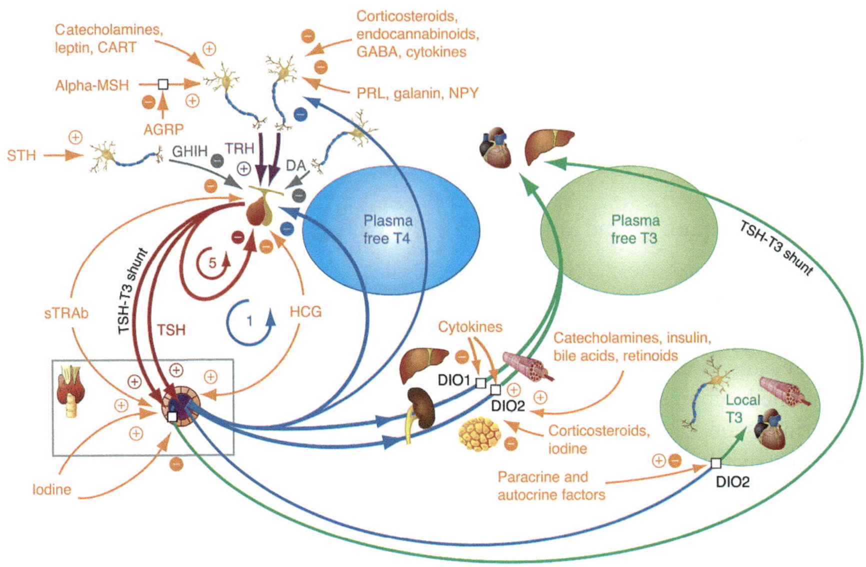

Fig. 5.1 Hypothalamic–pituitary–thyroid regulation
The hypothalamus, pituitary, and thyroid gland interact through a network of positive feed-forward (+) and negative feedback (−) loops. The respective hormones released by each gland into the circulation, namely TRH by the hypothalamus, TSH by the pituitary, and T4 and T3 by the thyroid gland, are involved in reciprocal (top–down and bottom–up) signalling between the glands. T3 is both synthesised de novo in the thyroid follicular cell and converted from T4 as a precursor by deiodinases. Both thyroidal processes are subject to TSH control (TSH feed-forward onto T3 or TSH-T3 shunt). The biological active free forms of T4 and T3, present in the circulation as small fractions of the protein-bound total hormones, are termed free T4 (FT4) and free T3 (FT3), respectively. Afferent signals project to the hypothalamus from higher brain centres. (The figure is adopted from Hoermann et al. [1])

thyroid and the pituitary gland [7]. Importantly, TSH and thyroid hormones assume *dual roles* in the homeostatic regulation, acting as controlling as well as controlled elements [8]. This establishes an intricate linkage between the controlling gland and the target gland [8–10]. Only a clear understanding and application of the principles of thyroid homeostasis provides in our view the necessary perspective for the diagnosis and treatment of thyroid dysfunction.

5.1 Homeostasis and Allostasis

Many challenges, often summarised under the term "stress" or "stressors", threaten the well-being or even survival of living organisms including humans, who must continuously cope with various types of stress in different situations. When adverse conditions arise outside the organism, the system must be able to protect its own inner environment and maintain a state of integrity and stability for the many dependent reactions. The property of the organism to resist stress and preserve a stable, relatively constant internal environment is generally known as *homeostasis* [11–14]. This is attained as an emergent property of a system or biochemical network, rather than a fixed target [15]. Maintenance of homeostasis typically involves the action of *negative feedback* mechanisms [16–18]. While defending the internal homeostatic state against stress is vital for the organism, it may not be sufficient in itself to adapt to rather adverse conditions as needed [19]. In the appropriate circumstances, it may be more advantageous for the system to show greater flexibility when adjusting to new demands, thereby moving away from its previous narrow homeostatic range to then adopt a new level of homeostasis [20, 21]. This brings *positive feedback* loops into play, which can amplify a variable of interest to shift the system from its previous homeostatic state to a new one [22, 23].

Together the mechanisms of control serve two opposing system properties [7]:

1. Robustness in resisting change to preserve the homeostatic state
2. Adaptation in supporting change to adjust the homeostatic state as required

The system must then decide which of the two options may be more advantageous in a given situation. The choice is either to withstand the stress by defending its current homeostatic level or to shift the homeostatic level to a new one which may better suit the altered conditions [7]. The *resilience* of a living system is expressed by choosing the most efficient path available, relying either on the mechanisms in support of the homeostasis or those in favour of its adaptation. It is this flexibility of the system in choosing the most appropriate response that reconciles the divisive concepts of homeostasis and allostasis [1, 24]. Both contribute to system stability and resilience as an overarching goal. To advance this perspective, it may be helpful to incorporate new concepts on the *free energy principle* and *self-organised criticality* into system regulation [14].

Extending the concept of homeostasis, the adaptive response of the system to stress which changes its previous homeostatic state has been termed *allostasis* [21, 24, 25]. Allostasis requires a more complex network of control involving both elements of top–down and bottom–up regulation to achieve the desired outcome [26]. The elements of *top–down* and *bottom–up* regulation in the hypothalamic–pituitary–thyroid (HPT) axis must be integrated in time and space to express the typical responses to varying stressors in thyroidal as well as non-thyroidal diseases [7]. This includes the accumulation of stress in the form of *allostatic load*, such as the history of memory effects and possible degeneration over time [24]. Crucially, top–down and bottom–up regulation extend to layers of feedback at levels above or below the next upstream or downstream level, because feedback and feed-forward loops merely at the next level are insufficient. In hypothalamic–pituitary–thyroid axis regulation negative feedback from thyroid (level 3) goes up to the next level, the pituitary (level 2) and the level after the next, the hypothalamus (level 1). Conversely, positive feed-forward comes down from the hypothalamus (level 1) to the next level, the pituitary (level 2), and the level after the next, the thyroid (level 3) (Fig. 5.1).

The *classical model* of hypothalamic–pituitary–thyroid (HPT) regulation is limited in its description to the pituitary control of the production of FT4 [1, 27, 28]. It does not give any consideration to other relevant feedback or feed-forward loops, particularly of feedback by thyroid hormones, neuronal afferences, tanycytes, and other humoral signals on TRH, and TSH feed-forward on FT3 generation (Fig. 5.1). As the classical model does not go beyond T4 production/supply, it cannot link thyroid hormone demand with supply to account for the utilisation of thyroid hormones appropriate for the metabolic needs of the various tissues in the body. By not considering these important properties otherwise, we came to the conclusion that our understanding of hypothalamic–pituitary–thyroid axis regulation *needs to be extended to include T3* [7]. The proper functioning of the hypothalamic–pituitary–thyroid axis is a prerequisite for the body to be able to meet its energetic needs. In particular, the *basal metabolic rate* and *resting energy expenditure* depend on the adequate supply and utilisation of thyroid hormones, a lack of which results in the hypothyroid disease spectrum. As a conclusion of our study, TSH and FT4 are not merely proportionally reflective of FT3 levels and the metabolic state of the individual but act jointly in a proactive way in the HPT axis regulation to stabilise FT3 levels and facilitate FT3 homeostasis/allostasis, as outlined in the concept of *relational stability* (see Chap. 2).

Anticipatory action is a key property of the regulatory system, with the system's defensive response preparing the organism for a perceived threat in advance without a prior need to experience the harmful impact on the body [7]. To this end, the control parameter, rather than being externally-driven, is controlled by the system itself, similar to the workings of a derivative control element in a technical proportional-integral-derivative (PID) controller [14]. This assumption appears to be consistent with the HPT axis regulation. By sensitivity analysis, we have shown that central T3 concentrations at the pituitary level, as opposed to T3 concentrations in the periphery, are upregulated by the activation of deiodinase type 2, allowing for the divergence in the central response from the peripheral equilibrium [29, 30]. The biochemical basis of this effect appears to be an *ubiquitination-dependent* mechanism unique to pituitary cells and different from that of peripheral cells expressing the same enzyme deiodinase type 2 [31]. Pituitary cells, unlike peripheral cells, increase the expression of the enzyme in the presence of high FT4 concentrations to maintain a high intracellular T3 level [31]. Also, the central nervous system, hypothalamus and pituitary gland express a specific thyroid hormone receptor (TRß2), with properties not shared by the peripheral thyroid hormone receptors, such as multiple contact coactivator recruitment, lack of activity without a ligand and enhanced sensitivity to thyroid hormones [32–34]. This may explain the pituitary's exceptionally sensitive response to a perceived thyroid function change in advance of the peripheral organs actually experiencing a hypothyroid state. The rational follows the free energy principle of minimising surprise and the fact that corrective preventive action is cost efficient, compared to later repair work [14]. In a simple analogy, you need to hit the brake, before you hit the car in front of you. Recent clinical studies agree with the model that TSH and FT4 cannot substitute for FT3 measurement. They equally refute a widely held belief, even among guidelines, that TSH always accurately represents the peripheral thyroid state [35, 36].

This is where the classical model becomes misleading by its limitations and falls short of correctly and accurately translating fundamental principles of hypothalamic–pituitary–thyroid axis regulation to the diagnosis and treatment of patients [7]. The actions of TSH in the greater T3-inclusive system of the HPT axis regulation are apparently designed to be corrective (proactive, adaptive), rather than reflective (post-hoc reactive). Addressing these issues in the next sections underpins and supports a necessary paradigm shift in patient care.

5.2 The Regulatory Network of the Hypothalamic–Pituitary–Thyroid Axis

Complex non-linear relationships between system components are operative in achieving a homeostatic state for a particular variable [1]. It follows that the behaviour of the complex network is *emergent and non-linear*, with sensitivities that are range-dependent. Sensitivity and variability at the higher levels tend to be greater, with the lower levels expressing greater simplicity, stability, and constancy. Change in the relationships between TSH and thyroid hormones or *relational stability* (see Chap. 2) must be considered when determining their physiologically and conditionally acceptable ranges in an individual [37]. As noted earlier, the dynamics and interrelations of these properties are not adequately reflected by the conventionally established and statistically derived population reference ranges for TSH, FT4, and FT3.

The regulatory hypothalamic–pituitary–thyroid network includes *three endocrine organs*, the hypothalamus, pituitary, and thyroid gland, and *four main hormones*, TRH, TSH, FT4, and FT3. The *interactions* between the glands and their specific hormones in space and time involve positive feed-forward mechanisms of the TRH input onto TSH, TSH input onto FT4, and TSH input onto FT3, and negative feedback mechanisms of FT4 input onto TSH and TRH and FT3 input onto TSH and TRH [1] (Fig. 5.1).

At the top level, the input of central brain signals activates the paraventricular nucleus of the hypothalamus. The afferences originate from the limbic system and other hypothalamic centres related to energy metabolism, with important modulating influences from, among others, tanycytes, cytokines, sex steroids, endocannabinoids, and glucocorticoids. These influences impact on the rate of synthesis and secretion of the hypothalamic hormone *TRH*. Thereby, TRH neurons together with neighbouring tanycytes become an important metabolic interface, the activity and interplay of these critical metabolic regulators being affected by variations in both internal and external environments [38–47]. Distinct subpopulations of hypophysiotropic TRH neurons may exist and respond to different stimuli, as has been suggested recently [48]. In addition, according to another novel discovery, TRH neurons have the ability to process T3 directly through axonal uptake and lysosomal transport [49]. *Tanycytes* are specialised glial cells located in proximity to TRH neurons.

They modulate the activity of the HPT axis by two TRH-dependent mechanisms, changes to the morphology of their endfeet that impede the vascular outflow of TRH and the expression of a TRH-degrading ectoenzyme [40, 50]. They express the deiodinase type 2 enzyme and are sensitive to thyroid hormones and other metabolic signals. TRH is released into the portal vein to be transported from the median eminence downstream to the pituitary gland. Arriving at the pituitary, it activates the local thyrotrophs (pituitary cells) to produce and release the pituitary hormone *TSH* into the circulation. When TSH, in turn, arrives at the thyroid gland and binds to its specific TSH receptor at the surface of the thyroid follicular cell, it enhances thyroidal hormone production, raising the low level of basal thyroid hormone secretion to that required for the metabolic needs of a healthy person. The thyroid releases mainly two hormones into the circulation, a *large amount of T4* and a *lesser amount of its sister hormone T3*. The latter is biologically more active than T4. It should be noted that glandular production is not the exclusive source of T3. T3 is additionally derived by *enzymatic T4 to T3 conversion* through monodeiodination [51]. In the blood stream, both T4 and T3 reversibly bind to thyroid hormone-binding proteins (TBG, transthyretin and albumin). Only a minute fraction of each hormone remains freely available, termed free T4 (FT4) and free T3 (FT3) [52]. The *free hormones* are the biologically active moieties. They are actively taken up by the various cells of the body using specific *transmembrane transporters* and reach their destination at the nucleus of the cell via further *intracellular transport* [53]. In the *nucleus*, specific DNA sites are responsive to T3 presented to them bound in a receptor complex. T3 exerts multiple actions at the gene level. Its *genomic actions* are classified as type 1 and type 2 signalling, according to Flamant et al. [54]. *Non-genomic T3 actions* are also known, but less well understood [55, 56]. The genomic actions of T3 induce both quantitative and qualitative changes in the expression of a multitude of gene products and proteins [57].

This means qualitative patterns differ between the euthyroid and hypothyroid state in a characteristic way. One example being the expression of a more energy-saving isotype of the enzyme *ATPase* in the heart muscle in hypothyroidism, compared to euthyroidism [58]. Accordingly, hypothyroidism must be regarded as a distinctly different qualitative and structural state from euthyroidism, not a mere quantitative extension of the euthyroid range [30]. A theoretical gland-mass model exploring the dynamics of thyroid disease and the complex inverse relation between TSH and FT4 supports the postulate of three regimes that stem from distinct clinical states of euthyroidism, hyperthyroidism and hypothyroidism [59]. This is reflected by *metabolonomics*, which reflects the differential regulation by thyroid states in their pattern of expression [60]. Successful treatment of hypothyroidism therefore involves a process of restructuring in a time frame appropriate for restoring the euthyroid state. This operates on a slower timescale than the biochemical "normalisation" of thyroid hormone concentrations, which precedes the structural recovery by months.

At the cell membrane and within the cell, various tissues, including the thyroid, express *different types of deiodinases* [31]. Consequently, T3, unlike T4, is not exclusively produced in the thyroid. In fact, in humans peripheral conversion of T4 to T3 is assumed to be the main source of T3, accounting for up to 80% of the total daily T3 production according to some authors [51]. However, there are several caveats to the assumption of this proportion. First, it relies on a few studies only. One frequently cited study was conducted by Pilo and colleagues [61]. However, others pointed out a high variability of these results depending on assumptions, ranging from 15% to 81% of the thyroidal T3 contribution [62]. Also, the fact that the participants were given high doses of iodine (Lugol solution)—acting as a blocker of thyroid hormone secretion and deiodination—may have led to substantial underestimation of the contribution of thyroidal T3 production to the T3 pool. Our studies suggest a significantly greater thyroidal T3 contribution and portray a more adaptive view of the hypothalamic–pituitary–thyroid axis regulation, including a provision of redundancy in the pathways and conditionally variable contributions by the thyroid to the circulating T3 pool [63, 64].

The thyroid gland finds itself at the forefront of the defence against a shortage of thyroid hormones. A greater importance of *glandular T3 secretion* in protecting FT3 concentrations emerges under conditions of diminished thyroid reserve as the thyroid strives to increase its own efficiency rather than solely relying on the increased productivity of other organs [64]. Of relevance, the reaction rates of the deiodinating enzymes in the thyroid and several other tissues are TSH-dependent [37, 65–70]. We may distinguish three *different sources* and mechanisms for the production of T3, namely

1. Largely T4-dependent, but TSH-independent T4 to T3 conversion in peripheral organs not expressing a functional TSH receptor
2. Both T4- and TSH-dependent T4 to T3 conversion in the thyroid and other organs that express a functional TSH receptor (e.g. brown adipose tissue)
3. T4-independent, but TSH-dependent T3 secretion by the thyroid

These mechanisms allow for *global and local adaptation* and tissue-specific modifications according to the individual needs of the different tissues, however, without granting them autonomy (total independence) from the central regulation [7]. Support of diversity is yet another important feature of the greater regulatory network of the hypothalamic–pituitary–thyroid axis regulation.

While FT4 exerts multiple genomic actions after its conversion to T3, non-genomic actions of T4 are also known, classified as type 3 and type 4 signalling [54, 71–73].

Insufficient concentrations of and/or responses to FT4 and FT3 are responsible for the disease spectrum of hypothyroidism, in essence an "energy deficiency" syndrome, while their excess leads to the diseases of thyrotoxicosis, an "energy excess" syndrome. Therefore, FT4 and FT3 must be kept in tight ranges for optimal functioning of the dependent reactions in the cells and organs of the body. FT4 and FT3 close negative feedback loops at the pituitary and hypothalamus by inhibiting the rate of production and secretion of the two upstream hormones, TSH and TRH (Fig. 5.1). The hormone concentration measured in the blood of a patient is the expression of the balance between the activating and repressing hormones, supporting the concept of relational stability in system regulation (Chap. 2). This concept describes the adaptive and range-dependent interrelations between the parameters that combine to support homeostasis and system stability.

In a clinical context, a measured TSH-FT4 pair is the conditionally intersecting point between the characteristic FT4 curve and the corresponding TSH curve [8, 74–76]. It indicates the *operating point* or *stable equilibrium* between TSH and FT4 in an individual at a given time. Traditionally, this is often called the *set point* of the pituitary–thyroid axis, as explained below. Notably, the very actions of TSH and FT4 that oppose each other in conditions of imminent thyroid failure combine in the integrated system of hypothalamic–pituitary–thyroid axis regulation and aim to protect FT3 homeostasis for as long as possible in these conditions [70].

5.3 The Functionality of the Hypothalamic–Pituitary–Thyroid Axis

Due to the complexity of the regulatory *hypothalamic–pituitary–thyroid system* (Fig. 5.1), mathematical models (Chap 4) have been used to generate testable hypotheses, predict the non-linear range-dependent responses to input signals and loads, and thereby inform about diagnostic and therapeutic procedures [1, 70].

5.3.1 TSH–FT4 Relationship

The *classical models* of pituitary thyrotropic feedback represent an early, yet simplistic and limited, description of pituitary–thyroid regulation [27, 77–79]. Nevertheless, these models linked observed behaviour to provide a phenomenological description of the relationship between the thyroid hormone FT4 and the pituitary hormone TSH [80]. Together with the advent of the development of highly sensitive assays for the measurement of TSH, this was instrumental in giving TSH its currently predominant role in clinical thyroid function testing [5].

Improved models later shifted to a parametrically isomorphic description, attempting to map results of physiological and molecular research to a cybernetic description of the information processing [74, 81, 82]. The history and evolvement of mathematical models of the hypothalamic–pituitary–thyroid axis regulation is beyond the scope of this book and has been reviewed elsewhere [1, 74]. More recent advances in mathematical modelling extended the perspective of control to the *greater hypothalamic–pituitary–thyroid system* beyond the TSH–FT4 relationship including FT3 homeostasis as an important goal of hypothalamic–pituitary–thyroid regulation [7]. The newer models have shown great potential, together with clinical studies, to shift our understanding of the role of TSH in the hypothalamic–pituitary–thyroid axis regulation formerly derived by the classical model, and appropriately redefine its clinical role to align it with the concept of relational stability (Chap. 2).

Despite their now recognised limitations, a brief review of the classical models may be warranted. Serious issues with this model will be addressed thereafter.

The classical model of thyroid homeostasis postulates a logarithmic relationship between FT4 levels and pituitary TSH release [83, 84]. Its advantage is a simple structure that allows for reconstructing the TSH–FT4 set point in open-loop situations [85]. In closed-loop analysis, the set point is at the intersection between the null isoclines of the feedback and feed-forward path in the equilibrium state. The mathematical deconstruction of the characteristic TSH and FT4 response curves of the pituitary and thyroid glands, respectively, enables the determination of this so-called set point [86]. The set point of an individual at a given time, measured as a pair of TSH and FT4 values in that person, is located at the intersection of the two characteristic curves, satisfying both conditions of the feed-forward and the feedback path [76]. Rather than using the term "set point", which is often misunderstood, the intersecting point should be more appropriately named a *balance point, operating point*, or *working point* under equilibrium conditions. The latter terms describe a flexibility in position according to need rather than an inflexibility which is rigidly enforced.

5.3.2 Attempts at Set Point Reconstruction

Population-derived *reference ranges* for thyrotropin and thyroid hormones are comparatively wide. They provide, therefore, a questionably accurate measure of *normality* and target for the dosage of substitution therapy. The working point (set point) of the feedback loop would define a more appropriate goal for dosage titration since it accounts for the central setting of the feedback loop and the individual sensitivity to thyroid hormone. However, in the state of hypothyroidism, it is impossible to know the location of the working point since neither the hypothalamic set point nor the thyroid response characteristics are known.

Methods of *set point reconstruction* rely on the following three assumptions:

- The working point of the feedback loop provides a suitable surrogate marker for the unobservable central set point.
- The pituitary response curve is basically unaltered in hypothyroidism.
- The working point is located in the vicinity of the largest curvature of the pituitary response curve, since this location ensures an optimal loop gain of the feedback control system.

According to the *MiMe-Log model* [75, 86], the characteristic response curves of the thyroid and pituitary can be described with the following defining equations [76].

The *response curve of the thyroid* to TSH is defined by

$$[FT_4] = \frac{K_T[TSH]}{D_T + [TSH]}$$

where K_T refers to a coefficient of the *maximum stimulated T4 secretion* (G_T) as estimated from the thyroid's secretory capacity for FT4 and relevant parameters of distribution, elimination, and plasma protein binding of T4, and DT is the *damping constant for TSH* at the pituitary.

The *response curve of the pituitary* to FT4 has to be inverted to enable the depiction of the TSH and FT4 curves in the same graph:

$$[TSH] = Se^{-\varphi[FT_4]}$$

where *S* refers to the intercept and phi to the gradient of the relationship.

The structural parameters *S* and phi can be empirically and individually estimated from a series of pairs of repeated TSH and FT4 measurements in an observed sample.

$$\varphi = \frac{1}{\left(FT_{4,1} - FT_{4,2}\right)} \ln \frac{TSH_1}{TSH_2}$$

$$S = TSH_1 e^{\varphi FT_{4,1}}$$

After logarithmic transformation, the response curves of the pituitary can be described as a log-linear TSH–FT4 relationship, with

$$\ln TSH = bFT_4 + c$$

where *b* refers to the slope of the logarithmic TSH curve and *c* its intercept with the *y* axis, with FT4 given in molar concentrations (pmol/L) and TSH in mIU/L.

Assuming that each individual has its own defining structural parameters, such as a maximum thyroid capacity (G_T) and its derived coefficient K_T, maximum pituitary capacity (*S*) and a fixed trajectory for the gradient of the TSH–FT4 relationship (phi), and that the fixpoint of the feedback loop is located in the vicinity of the maximum curvature of the pituitary response curve, which yields an optimal loop gain, we can create individual trajectories for the FT4 response curve and inverted TSH response curve, as shown in Fig. 5.2. In Fig. 5.2, the levels of the maximum thyroid capacity (GT = 1.67, 3.43 or 7.51 pmol/s) and derived KT were chosen so as to correspond to the average and 95% confidence interval typical of a clinical study in thyroid-healthy subjects [87]. The pituitary response curves shown share the same maximum pituitary response (intercept *S* = 200), and vary in their gradient (phi = 0.3 or 0.5). The *intersections* of the two curves each define an individually observable balance point or the so-called set point. In a population, the observable set points of the individuals are *clustered*.

We note that the reconstruction of individual set points (working points) derived from repeated measurements of the TSH–FT4 pairs over time can be expected to deliver an improved and more personalised solution, compared to the population-based statistics that are currently used for defining the reference ranges for thyroid hormones and TSH [75, 86]. Importantly, the shape of the reference range of a more realistic bivariate and clustered approach forms a *kite-shaped area* [74, 76] but does not enclose a rectangle, such as the conventional reference range, which considers the

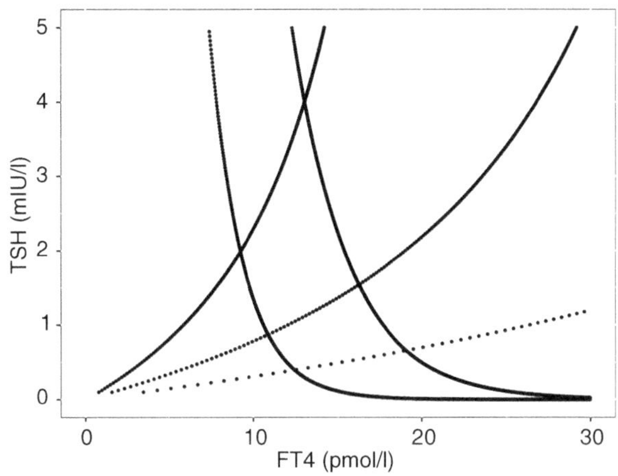

Fig. 5.2 Set point (working point) reconstruction
The FT4 curve moves from left to right with increasing TSH values driving FT4 levels up. Three FT4 curves are shown, depending on functional thyroid capacity (GT), representing its 2.5th, 50th and 97.5th percentile in healthy subjects. The TSH curve moves downward as FT4 levels increase. The two TSH curves approximate the 2.5th and 97.5th percentiles of healthy subjects. The working point (also called the set point) is found at the intersection between a corresponding TSH and FT4 curve. The 95% bivariate reference range is the kite-shaped area enclosed by the four outer intersecting points. In contrast, the conventionally used separate reference ranges for each hormone form a rectangle. For details see text; for code to produce the curves refer to Supplement of [76]

two hormones separately, each with a univariable distribution. Clinical disease classifications particularly of subclinical hypothyroidism differ substantially, based on the different techniques used to derive the respective ranges of reference and normality. Lacking a clinical definition of subclinical disease and relying solely on conventional laboratory ranges currently pose a substantial dilemma for clinicians particularly when deciding on thresholds and targets for the required treatment [88, 89]. *Calculated parameters* and relationships have emerged as novel tools in clinical research [90]. Set point computation has been proposed for personalised dosing to improve and individualise thyroid hormone replacement with levothyroxine [86]. On a note of caution, although these techniques offer improvements over the use of conventional population-based reference ranges towards individualisation of patient care, they fall short of a more complete and FT3-inclusive perspective, which has been derived from mathematical modelling of the hypothalamic–pituitary–thyroid axis regulation [7].

5.3.3 FT3 Homeostasis as a System Goal

Fixed reference points and ranges, as desirable as they may be, systematically disregard the effects of altered equilibria and can thereby introduce considerable bias when interpreting TSH measurements for diagnostic use. This has already been discussed earlier when introducing the concept of *relational stability* (Chap. 2).

As our basic understanding of the complex regulatory mechanisms in the hypothalamic–pituitary–thyroid control has evolved, the following major fundamental concerns have emerged from recent theoretical and clinical studies that need to be addressed to improve the current standard of patient care [70].

1. The *disruption of homeostatic mechanisms* leads to disease and makes it essential for the therapy to be effective to aim at restoring the homeostatic conditions [13].
2. Thyroid parameters display a high degree of *individuality*, with each patient having their own characteristic structural parameters that are partly genetically determined and striving to maintain much narrower personal optima at variable distances from the population's average [6, 91, 92].
3. The *conditionality* of the equilibria displaces "normal" ranges, which are for instance different in LT4-treated patients, compared to those in healthy controls [37].
4. The concept of relational stability (see Chap. 2) emphasizes the role of the combined actions of TSH and FT4 for the maintenance of FT3 homeostasis. This is particularly relevant in the event of early thyroid failure. It works through the appropriate adaption of the relationships still within the euthyroid range or extending into the range of subclinical hypothyroidism [37].

An understanding of the latter issues and their consequences requires the incorporation of the biologically more active thyroid hormone FT3 into *a more complete view* on the system of hypothalamic–pituitary–thyroid axis regulation and the design of an *extended model*. Both the complexity of the regulatory network (Fig. 5.1) and the apparent limitations of the TSH–FT4 perspective (classical model) and set point theory made it desirable to extend the concept of hypothalamic–pituitary–thyroid axis regulation beyond the phenomenological TSH–FT4 relationship in order to integrate the more active sister hormone FT3 and *mechanisms of FT3 homeostasis* into the systemic regulation [7, 70]. This approach elevates the role of FT3 and its homeostasis to a system goal. It contrasts with the current guidelines for the diagnosis and treatment of hypothyroidism that give little, if any, consideration to FT3 determination. On the contrary, FT3 measurements have been declared redundant and are currently not endorsed by guidelines, which recommend measurements of TSH and FT4 only [5].

This in our opinion erroneous view on the role of FT3 is based on three *mistaken assumptions*:

1. A subnormal assessment of FT4 establishes the diagnosis of hypothyroidism, and TSH is exquisitely sensitive to minor changes in FT4. This led to the adoption of TSH as the single best screening test for primary hypothyroidism and the definition of biochemically subclinical hypothyroidism in the absence of both clinical symptoms and low FT4 concentrations [5].
2. T4 is always converted to T3 as needed, leading to the redundancy of FT3 measurement and a change in the treatment mode of hypothyroidism to levothyroxine only replacement.

3. TSH within its reference range represents the most accurate marker of euthyroidism, guiding both the diagnosis of hypothyroidism and its treatment, particularly the adjustment of levothyroxine dosage, so as to return TSH within its normal range.

All three assumptions have long been challenged by reported patients' experience and multiple clinical studies [29, 35, 36, 93, 94]. They have now also been strongly refuted and superseded by more advanced FT3-inclusive mathematical modelling of the hypothalamic–pituitary–thyroid axis regulation [7, 70]. These advanced models demand a fundamental re-evaluation of the role of FT3 in the context of homeostatic considerations and the physiologically complex system of the hypothalamic–pituitary–thyroid axis regulation.

5.3.4 Attainment of FT3 Homeostasis

Perfect FT3 homeostasis can be mathematically defined as a near constancy of FT3 levels when the FT4 and TSH concentrations change substantially, for instance when the T4 production rate changes over a wide range in the transition from normal thyroid function to thyroid failure in hypothyroidism. A brief introduction to *mathematical modelling* is provided in Chap. 4. This allows a more fundamental theoretical investigation into the clinically observable concept of *relational stability* (Chap. 2) using a mathematical modelling approach [7].

We examined the interaction of the constitutive loops of the hypothalamic–pituitary–thyroid axis regulation. They consist of positive feed-forward of TRH influence onto TSH, TSH influence onto FT4 and FT3, and negative feedback loops of FT4 and FT3 influences onto TSH and TRH (Fig. 5.3). This study revealed that despite the complexity of the system it is possible to readily attain a solution of perfect FT3 homeostasis under these conditions.

When *normalising* the strengths of the interacting loops, setting them to 1 (100%), and also keeping other parameters and removal rates constant at 1, this regulatory system achieves perfect FT3 homeostasis in the presence of changing FT4 and TSH concentrations. In this case, expressing a constant stable FT3 equilibrium solution of square root of 2 (Fig. 5.4).

The FT3 solution that emerges is surprisingly simple, given the complexity of this system. This means that the hypothalamic–pituitary–thyroid axis regulation is capable of monitoring and filtering diverse influences at the top end and aggregating their input. The information is processed through the system and the signal is transferred downwards to fine-tune the response with high precision and accuracy. *Flexibility at the upper end translates into stability at the lower end*, combining *robustness in performance* with *precision in adaptation* [7].

We note the *complexity* of natural systems seemingly precludes simplified implications in the quantitative analysis of disease states. However, the argument weakens and simplification may be permitted, at least to some extent, because complex

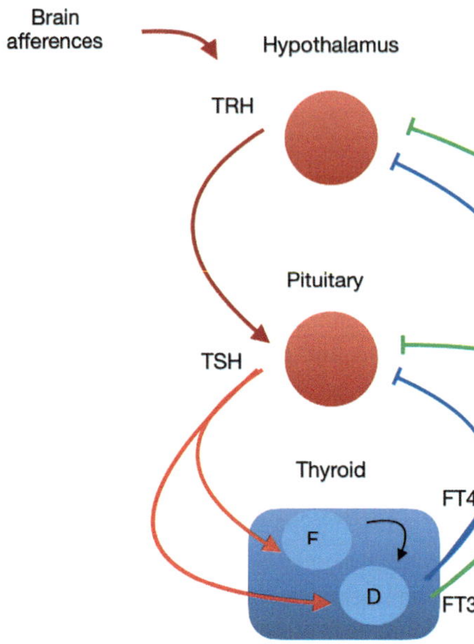

Fig. 5.3 Interactive loops of hypothalamic–pituitary–thyroid regulation
The hypothalamus is activated by higher brain centres. Hypothalamic TRH activates pituitary TSH, and TSH activates thyroidal T4 and T3 production. T4 and T3 are synthesised in thyroid follicles (F). T4 is converted to T3 by TSH-dependent deiodinases (D). Circulating free forms of T4 and T3 are FT4 and FT3, respectively. The loops are closed by FT4 and FT3 repressing TSH and TRH production

pathways can often be dealt with as *aggregates* of input/output monotone subsystems, allowing different chain elements to be combined into a single element, as demonstrated here. We have also demonstrated high congruence between our minimal proof-of-concept model and a fully parametrised model [70]. Of note, when modelling regulation of thyroid function, our model assumed iodine sufficiency to allow for proper gland function. This model does not address the pathophysiology of iodine deficiency disorders and euthyroid goitre. A comprehensive model of 22 compartments including a sub-model of iodine metabolism has for instance been described by Pompa et al. [95].

The FT3-homeostatic mechanisms in the hypothalamic–pituitary–thyroid regulation present an accomplished example of the general utility of *paradoxical components*, among other incomplete feed-forward loops, in the design of biological circuits [96]. Such components render the concentrations of the end product of the system response independent of possible variations in the availability of its precursor [96]. Apparently, this is an inherent physiological system property expressed by the core system of the hypothalamic–pituitary–thyroid axis [7]. Thereby, the coordinated movements of FT4 and TSH in opposite directions help stabilise FT3

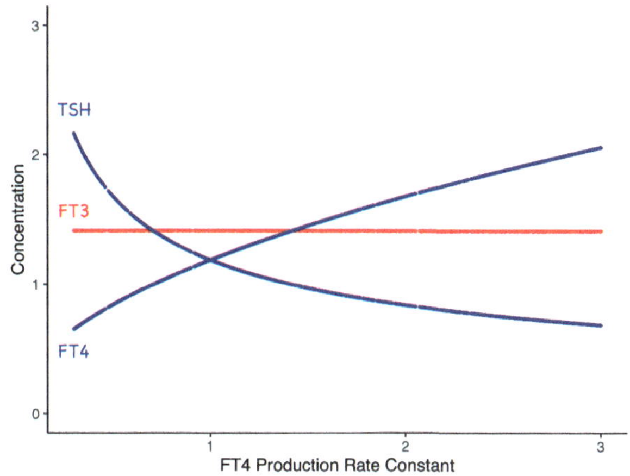

Fig. 5.4 Demonstration of attainment of perfect FT3 homeostasis in hypothalamic–pituitary–thyroid axis regulation in a mathematical model
The interactive loops of the hypothalamic–pituitary–thyroid axis regulation (Fig. 5.3) enable the actions of TRH (not shown), TSH, and FT4 to cooperate in a way to produce an equilibrium solution of perfect homeostasis for FT3 (horizontal line at 1.41, square root of 2). This is an example of relational stability. The strengths of all limbs have been normalised. For further details see text, and for the mathematical solution and code to create the figure refer to [7]

concentrations and *preserve FT3 homeostasis*. Neither of the levels of the two other hormones is therefore directly reflective of the FT3 levels, rather both interact to achieve and maintain FT3 homeostasis in the normal thyroid state [7].

This behaviour redefines the role of TSH as a controlling element and *corrective agent*, rather than an accurate marker always reflective of the euthyroid state [70]. This substantially changes the classical system perspective (Table 5.1). Consequently, the *roles of TSH* in defining euthyroidism and hypothyroidism are separated. TSH is a sensitive indicator of a shortage in thyroid hormone supply, particularly in primary hypothyroidism, making it a valuable asset in the diagnosis of overt primary hypothyroidism. However, the importance of TSH diminishes towards the euthyroid range, where it loses discriminatory accuracy and prognostic value, because here it is corrective, but uncorrelated to the underlying thyroid status and also much more variable between subjects [92].

Subclinical hypothyroidism as defined by TSH elevation and within-reference range FT4 concentrations is an intermediate state of uncertain functionality in terms of true hypothyroidism or euthyroidism. It can be regarded as *stressed euthyroid syndrome* and may fall in either diagnostic category, euthyroid or hypothyroid, depending or whether or not TSH correction has been successful, particularly in restoring FT3 homeostasis in early thyroid failure [87].

Apart from indicating possible early thyroid failure (capacity stress), a moderate rise in TSH is also part of the general stress response of the organism. This

Table 5.1 System perspective of thyroid hormones

Classical system perspective	Extended system perspective
System is limited to pituitary–thyroid regulation	System extends to hypothalamic–pituitary–thyroid regulation
Main hormones involved are TSH and FT4	Main hormones involved are FT3, FT4, TSH, TRH
Negative feedback by FT4 on TSH and feed-forward of TSH on FT4	Network of multiple feedback and feed-forward loops over several hierarchies and hormones
TSH supports FT4 homeostasis	TSH and FT4 support FT3 homeostasis
TSH reflects the peripheral thyroid state	TSH is designed to correct the peripheral thyroid state
TSH is reactive	TSH is anticipatory
TSH gains precedence over FT4	FT3 gains precedence over TSH and FT4
FT3 has no role in the system	FT3 is integrated into the system
Isolated interpretation of each hormone	Joined interpretation of hormones
Health depends on concentrations of hormones within reference range	Health depends on relational stability between hormones

introduces yet another ambiguity and statistical conflation in the current definition of subclinical hypothyroidism [97]. The latter situation has nothing to do with the functionality of the thyroid gland per se. These particularities in the hypothalamic–pituitary–thyroid axis regulation explain why a formal biochemical diagnosis of subclinical hypothyroidism according to the guidelines is insufficient for the treatment decision. As a consequence, the same criteria and consistent thresholds do not equally apply to the diagnosis and treatment of hypothyroidism. The latter can become rather confusing to clinicians and patients alike.

The separation of the diagnosis of a "disease" from its requirement of treatment is a cause of considerable misunderstanding between patients and physicians [88]. The inadequate disease understanding promoted by current guidelines has left clinicians with a conundrum to explain to many patients why they suffer from a disease, yet would not require any therapeutic intervention. Many clinicians therefore regard the term of "subclinical hypothyroidism" for the description of a TSH-dominated laboratory constellation as a misnomer. Perhaps the time has come to find a more accurate and clinically inclusive definition for "subclinical thyroid disease", more deserving of this name [89].

5.3.5 Clinical Implications of a FT3-Inclusive Perspective

Integration of FT3 homeostasis in the hypothalamic–pituitary–thyroid axis regulation changes the physiological perspective and clinical interpretation of this system in important ways [70]:

1. Hypothalamic–pituitary–thyroid axis regulation provides *FT3-homeostatic mechanisms*, particularly through a FT3-TSH shunt and a TSH-feed-forward motif onto the production of FT3 (relational stability).
2. FT3 concentrations move *non-proportionally* to FT4 and TSH, being still homeostatically maintained when the other two hormones may vary substantially and, in fact, attained through the coordinated variation of the other two hormones (Fig. 5.4).
3. FT3 concentrations are *insensitive* to a moderate change in thyroid function. An increase in TSH is supportive of FT3 homeostasis, acting as a protective mechanism to restore or adapt FT3 homeostasis and avoid disease-related symptoms in early thyroid failure for as long as possible.
4. The *corrective actions* of TSH in supporting FT3 homeostasis dissociate the measurement of its concentration from merely passively reflecting the underlying euthyroid state in a patient. For that reason, TSH cannot serve as an invariably reliable indicator of euthyroidism.
5. It follows that *TSH "normalisation"* within its reference range is not an accurate measure of treatment success and dose adequacy in patients on levothyroxine replacement.
6. *Measurement of FT3* is required in patient care and useful in its own right, in addition to TSH and FT4.
7. *FT3 homeostasis* aims to maintain the energetic and metabolic needs of the organism. It is subject to and integrated with central control, notwithstanding additional local mechanisms of adaption and diversity.
8. *Interconnected complex networks* as expressed by the hypothalamic–pituitary–thyroid axis jointly express mechanisms of homeostasis and allostasis for optimum resilience.
9. FT3 *upregulates* deiodinase type 1 activity (Table 3.3), thereby facilitating T4 to T3 conversion in liver, kidney, and thyroid.
10. Hypothyroidism as a disease should be defined more comprehensively as a *failure of supply and/or utilisation of thyroid hormones*, reintroducing a previous definition found in older text books.
11. Disregarding the *distinct roles of FT3* in hypothalamic–pituitary–thyroid regulation as in patients on levothyroxine monotherapy is predicted to cause issues of symptomatic relief (Chap. 8).

5.3.6 Anticipation as a System Property

The regulatory network of the hypothalamic–pituitary–thyroid axis displays several *essential properties* at the system level [7]. This system combines *robustness* in performance with *adaptivity* in its responsiveness to stressors, as already explained. An awareness of a potential threat *in advance* of the actual event defines a desirable system property. Anticipatory action and a defensive response of the system prepare the organism for an imminent risk in advance of the actual experience of harm. In the hypothalamic–pituitary–thyroid axis regulation, thyroid hormones stored in the thyroid follicles are provisioned and utilised without immediately affecting FT3 utilisation and disrupting the FT3-dependent energetic and metabolic processes in the body. The anticipatory mechanisms of the regulatory system are designed to *maintain FT3 homeostasis* over a considerable range independently of thyroidal T4 production. They can also rely on direct glandular T3 secretion as a complementary and adjustable pathway [64]. This requires the pituitary TSH response to be extraordinarily sensitive, act correctively, and its actions to precede the manifestation of hypothyroidism. For that reason, the use of TSH and FT4 measurements as surrogates of FT3 is denied [36]. Evidently, this property of the hypothalamic–pituitary–thyroid system regulation conflicts with the widely held belief of pituitary TSH reflecting the euthyroid state as an accurate marker. Of note, *superior sensitivity* required for needed or anticipated correction must not be confused with high accuracy in defining the underlying thyroid state in the clinical interpretation of thyroid function testing.

5.3.7 Ultradian and Circadian Rhythms of TSH and Thyroid Hormone Secretion

Another example of anticipatory provisioning is the *seasonal pattern* found in the responsiveness of the hypothalamic–pituitary–thyroid system [98]. This phenomenon has been described in many animal species, including, to a lesser extent, in humans [99]. One uncovered intricate mechanism, among others, involves a *variant form of TSH* that is produced in the pars tibialis of the pituitary gland and termed ptTSH [100, 101]. This hormone is functionally different from TSH, devoid of thyroid-stimulating activity and sensitive to melatonin. Unlike the thyroid, both TRH neurons and neighbouring tanycytes respond to ptTSH. Depending on the season, as reflected by the length of day light and melatonin concentrations, ptTSH adjusts the TRH input to the hypothalamic–pituitary–thyroid axis regulation. The signal is translated downstream to adapt the level of FT3 homeostasis accordingly. Concomitant to the functional activation of the regulatory cascade, thyroid growth is also promoted to increase the *gland mass* [98]. This *sensitises* the thyroid towards TSH stimulation, inducing the release of a greater amount of thyroid hormone(s) per unit of TSH. The increase in circulating thyroid hormone concentrations, in turn, leads to the suppression and shrinkage of the pituitary. This process induces a *cyclical pattern* of growth and gland mass regulation between the thyroid and pituitary [98]. Because the space in the sella turcica where the human pituitary resides is limited, the proliferation of thyrotrophs also involves the recruitment and *specialisation* of other pituitary cells. This refutes a former hypothesis associating each specialised pituitary cell type with the secretion of a single pituitary hormone. Seasonal variations in serum TSH levels and thyroid hormones have been documented in clinical studies [99]. Moreover, a seasonal pattern in the concentrations of circulating thyroid hormones has been retained even in patients treated for hypothyroidism with levothyroxine [102].

Like other *glycoprotein hormones*, TSH is secreted in a *pulsatile* manner [103, 104]. Faster *oscillations* with a mean pulse amplitude of 0.6 mIU/l and a rate of 5–20/24 h are superimposed on a circadian rhythm with maximum TSH levels shortly after midnight. The origin of the observed oscillations is still debated. The notion that fast TSH pulses emerge as a function of pulsatile TRH input has been contradicted by some authors [105]. Other possibilities include stochastic signals or autocrine function of thyrotrophs, partly emanating from ultrashort feedback [82]. TSH pulsatility may be beneficial by preventing homologous desensitisation of the thyrotropin receptor. This could partly explain why sialylated TSH has both prolonged half-life and reduced bioactivity [106]. TSH-feed-forward and its deiodinase links may be to some extent responsible for the circadian rhythm of FT3 accompanying that of TSH, while FT4 concentrations show no such circadian rhythm [107]. In severe thyroid dysfunction, the response was experimentally modulated by regulating TSH receptor density [108]. All these mechanisms align the task of maintaining and adapting FT3 homeostasis with the central control system. This, in turn, may have served a higher goal of energy allocation in a way that was advantageous for human evolution [21].

Clinically, *physiological variations* of the hormone level over the course of the day have to be considered when using TSH measurements for diagnostic purposes. For optimal *comparability* between different measurements, blood sample should best be obtained at the same time in the morning and before the intake of any thyroid medication [109].

5.3.8 Memory Effects and Hysteresis

Gland size regulation of the pituitary and thyroid, along with their functional control in the hypothalamic–pituitary–thyroid axis regulation, directly changes the sensitivity of the thyroid to TSH [59]. Both gland functions and the sizes of the controlling and target organs appear to be generally *linked* and proportional [8, 10]. This can be viewed as an expression of structure–function relationship. It is involved in the expression of observable *seasonality* in the system response, as described above. As the mechanisms of gland mass control operate on a slower timescale, compared to the more rapid regulation of thyroid function, the *lagging response* between the two modes of control produces an inherent memory effect of the past [59]. This phenomenon is commonly known as *hysteresis* effect.

Clinically, this means that a given TSH–FT4 relationship is not fixed and invariant in time. Rather it may display a *hysteresis* phenomenon where the current system response still remains influenced by past events in the history of the patient (Fig. 5.5).

As an example, long-standing suppression of TSH under levothyroxine medication may lead to pituitary atrophy. A dose reduction of the levothyroxine drug may

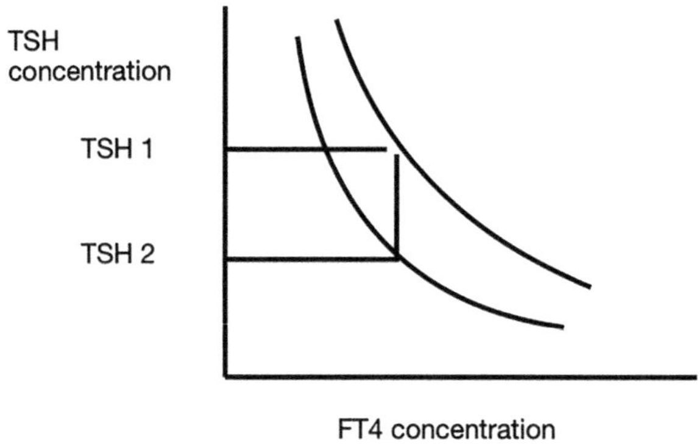

Fig. 5.5 Hysteresis effect
The TSH-FT4 trajectories show a delay possibly causing a hysteresis effect for TSH concentrations relative to the FT4 concentrations for instance in a patient with autoimmune thyroiditis. Such a memory effect may be explained by a gland mass model according to [59]

then fail to trigger a rise in the TSH level, otherwise expected. The measured TSH value is still *linked to the past* condition instead of indicating the current altered situation [110].

Timing and possible *non-equilibrium* of TSH measurements have to be clinically considered when ordering thyroid function tests. Any change in thyroid hormone production or exogenous thyroid hormone supply is typically accompanied by a delay of 4–8 weeks for the TSH response to reach a stable equilibrium. Not considering the possibility of a hysteresis effect in such situations may lead to clinical misdiagnosis and false treatment decisions.

The TSH molecule may further undergo *qualitative change* in its glycosylation depending on thyroid function, which, in turn, can modify both its *bioactivity* and the ratio of its immunological to biological activity [111].

References

1. Hoermann R, Midgley JEM, Larisch R, Dietrich JW. Homeostatic control of the thyroid-pituitary axis: perspectives for diagnosis and treatment. Front Endocrinol (Lausanne). 2015;6:177. https://doi.org/10.3389/fendo.2015.00177.
2. Caldwell G, Kellett HA, Gow SM, Beckett GJ, Sweeting VM, Seth J, Toft AD. A new strategy for thyroid function testing. Lancet. 1985;1:1117–9.
3. Baloch Z, Carayon P, Conte-Devolx B, Demers LM, Feldt-Rasmussen U, Henry JF, Livosli VA, Niccoli-Sire P, John R, Ruf J, Smyth PP, Spencer CA, Stockigt JR, Guidelines Committee NAOCB. Laboratory medicine practice guidelines. Laboratory support for the diagnosis and monitoring of thyroid disease. Thyroid. 2004;13:3–126. https://doi.org/10.1089/105072503321086962.
4. Spencer CA. Laboratory thyroid tests: a historical perspective. Thyroid. 2023;33:407–19. https://doi.org/10.1089/thy.2022.0397.

5. Jonklaas J, Bianco AC, Bauer AJ, Burman KD, Cappola AR, Celi FS, Cooper DS, Kim BW, Peeters RP, Rosenthal MS, Sawka AM. Guidelines for the treatment of hypothyroidism: prepared by the American Thyroid Association task force on thyroid hormone replacement. Thyroid. 2014;24:1670–751. https://doi.org/10.1089/thy.2014.0028.
6. Midgley JEM, Toft AD, Larisch R, Dietrich JW, Hoermann R. Time for a reassessment of the treatment of hypothyroidism. BMC Endocr Disord. 2019;19:37. https://doi.org/10.1186/s12902-019-0365-4.
7. Hoermann R, Pekker M, Midgley JEM, Larisch R, Dietrich JW. Principles of endocrine regulation: reconciling tensions between robustness in performance and adaptation to change. Front Endocrinol (Lausanne). 2022;13:825107. https://doi.org/10.3389/fendo.2022.825107.
8. Fitzgerald SP, Bean NG, Falhammar H, Hoermann R. Physiological linkage of thyroid and pituitary sensitivities. Endocrine. 2023;79:143–51. https://doi.org/10.1007/s12020-022-03184-8.
9. Fitzgerald SP, Bean NG, Falhammar H, Hoermann R, Korem Kohanim Y, Pohlabeln H, Grote Beverborg N, Tomassetti S. Population data evidence of interdependence of the limbs of hormonal feedback loops. J Endocrinol. 2024;262:e230384. https://doi.org/10.1530/JOE-23-0384.
10. Raz M, Milo T, Glass DS, Mayo A, Alon U. Endocrine gland size is proportional to its target tissue size. iScience. 2024;27(9):110625. https://doi.org/10.1016/j.isci.2024.110625.
11. Cannon WB, Rosenberg CE. Homeostasis. The wisdom of the body. New York: Norton; 1932.
12. Lu X, Jin G, Chen W, Yu X, Ling F. Depiction of physiological homeostasis by self-coupled system and its significance. Front Physiol. 2019;10:1205. https://doi.org/10.3389/fphys.2019.01205.
13. Billman GE. Homeostasis: the underappreciated and far too often ignored central organizing principle of physiology. Front Physiol. 2020;11:200. https://doi.org/10.3389/fphys.2020.00200.
14. Bettinger JS, Friston KJ. Conceptual foundations of physiological regulation incorporating the free energy principle and self-organized criticality. Neurosci Biobehav Rev. 2023;155:105459. https://doi.org/10.1016/j.neubiorev.2023.105459.
15. Golubitsky M, Stewart I, Antoneli F, Huang Z, Wang Y. Input-output networks, singularity theory, and homeostasis. Advances in dynamics, optimization and computation. In: Proceedings of the workshop on dynamics, optimization and computation held in honor of the 60th birthday of Michael Dellnitz; 2020. p. 31–65. https://doi.org/10.1007/978-3-030-51264-4_2.
16. Sauro HM. Control and regulation of pathways via negative feedback. J R Soc Interface. 2017;14:20160848. https://doi.org/10.1098/rsif.2016.0848.
17. Reed M, Best J, Golubitsky M, Stewart I, Nijhout HF. Analysis of homeostatic mechanisms in biochemical networks. Bull Math Biol. 2017;79:2534–57. https://doi.org/10.1007/s11538-017-0340-z.
18. Nijhout HF, Best JA, Reed MC. Systems biology of robustness and homeostatic mechanisms. Wiley Interdiscip Rev Syst Biol Med. 2019;11:e1440. https://doi.org/10.1002/wsbm.1440.
19. Sterling P. What is health?: allostasis and the evolution of human design. Cambridge, MA: MIT Press; 2020. p. 1–225.
20. Hoermann R, Midgley JEM, Larisch R, Dietrich JW. Recent advances in thyroid hormone regulation: toward a new paradigm for optimal diagnosis and treatment. Front Endocrinol (Lausanne). 2017;8:364. https://doi.org/10.3389/fendo.2017.00364.
21. Levy SB, Bribiescas RG. Hierarchies in the energy budget: thyroid hormones and the evolution of human life history patterns. Evol Anthropol. 2023;32:275–92. https://doi.org/10.1002/evan.22000.
22. Cinquin O, Demongeot J. Roles of positive and negative feedback in biological systems. C R Biol. 2002;325:1085–95. https://doi.org/10.1016/S1631-0691(02)01533-0.
23. Pfeuty B, Kaneko K. The combination of positive and negative feedback loops confers exquisite flexibility to biochemical switches. Phys Biol. 2009;6:046013. https://doi.org/10.1088/1478-3975/6/4/046013.

24. Chatzitomaris A, Hoermann R, Midgley JEM, Hering S, Urban A, Dietrich B, Abood A, Klein HH, Dietrich JW. Thyroid allostasis-adaptive responses of thyrotropic feedback control to conditions of strain, stress, and developmental programming. Front Endocrinol (Lausanne). 2017;8:163. https://doi.org/10.3389/fendo.2017.00163.
25. Sterling P. Principles of allostasis: optimal design, predictive regulation, pathophysiology and rational therapeutics. In: Schulkin J, editor. Allostasis, homeostasis, and the costs of physiological adaptation. Cambridge University Press; 2003. p. 1–36.
26. Rauss K, Pourtois G. What is bottom-up and what is top-down in predictive coding. Front Psychol. 2013;4:276. https://doi.org/10.3389/fpsyg.2013.00276.
27. Reichlin S, Utiger RD. Regulation of the pituitary-thyroid axis in man: relationship of TSH concentration to concentration of free and total thyroxine in plasma. J Clin Endocrinol Metab. 1967;27:251–5. https://doi.org/10.1210/jcem-27-2-251.
28. Larsen PR. Thyroid-pituitary interaction: feedback regulation of thyrotropin secretion by thyroid hormones. N Engl J Med. 1982;306:23–32. https://doi.org/10.1056/NEJM198201073060107.
29. Hoermann R, Midgley JEM, Larisch R, Dietrich JW. Is pituitary TSH an adequate measure of thyroid hormone-controlled homoeostasis during thyroxine treatment. Eur J Endocrinol. 2013;168:271–80. https://doi.org/10.1530/EJE-12-0819.
30. Midgley JEM, Hoermann R, Larisch R, Dietrich JW. Physiological states and functional relation between thyrotropin and free thyroxine in thyroid health and disease: in vivo and in silico data suggest a hierarchical model. J Clin Pathol. 2013;66:335–42. https://doi.org/10.1136/jclinpath-2012-201213.
31. Gereben B, Zavacki AM, Ribich S, Kim BW, Huang SA, Simonides WS, Zeöld A, Bianco AC. Cellular and molecular basis of deiodinase-regulated thyroid hormone signaling. Endocr Rev. 2008;29:898–938. https://doi.org/10.1210/er.2008-0019.
32. Langlois MF, Zanger K, Monden T, Safer JD, Hollenberg AN, Wondisford FE. A unique role of the beta-2 thyroid hormone receptor isoform in negative regulation by thyroid hormone. Mapping of a novel amino-terminal domain important for ligand-independent activation. J Biol Chem. 1997;272:24927–33.
33. Wan W, Farboud B, Privalsky ML. Pituitary resistance to thyroid hormone syndrome is associated with T3 receptor mutants that selectively impair beta2 isoform function. Mol Endocrinol. 2005;19:1529–42. https://doi.org/10.1210/me.2005-0014.
34. Lee S, Young BM, Wan W, Chan IH, Privalsky ML. A mechanism for pituitary-resistance to thyroid hormone (prth) syndrome: a loss in cooperative coactivator contacts by thyroid hormone receptor (tr)beta2. Mol Endocrinol. 2011;25:1111–25. https://doi.org/10.1210/me.2010-0448.
35. Fitzgerald SP, Bean NG, Falhammar H, Tuke J. Clinical parameters are more likely to be associated with thyroid hormone levels than with thyrotropin levels: a systematic review and meta-analysis. Thyroid. 2020;30:1695–709. https://doi.org/10.1089/thy.2019.0535.
36. Lawton RI, Sabatini BL, Hochbaum DR. Longevity, demographic characteristics, and socio-economic status are linked to triiodothyronine levels in the general population. Proc Natl Acad Sci USA. 2024;121:e2308652121. https://doi.org/10.1073/pnas.2308652121.
37. Hoermann R, Midgley JEM, Larisch R, Dietrich JW. Relational stability in the expression of normality, variation, and control of thyroid function. Front Endocrinol (Lausanne). 2016;7:142. https://doi.org/10.3389/fendo.2016.00142.
38. Lechan RM, Fekete C. The TRH neuron: a hypothalamic integrator of energy metabolism. Prog Brain Res. 2006;153:209–35. https://doi.org/10.1016/S0079-6123(06)53012-2.
39. López M, Alvarez CV, Nogueiras R, Diéguez C. Energy balance regulation by thyroid hormones at central level. Trends Mol Med. 2013;19:418–27. https://doi.org/10.1016/j.molmed.2013.04.004.
40. Müller-Fielitz H, Stahr M, Bernau M, Richter M, Abele S, Krajka V, Benzin A, Wenzel J, Kalies K, Mittag J, Heuer H, Offermanns S, Schwaninger M. Tanycytes control the hormonal

output of the hypothalamic-pituitary-thyroid axis. Nat Commun. 2017;8:484. https://doi.org/10.1038/s41467-017-00604-6.
41. Tran LT, Park S, Kim SK, Lee JS, Kim KW, Kwon O. Hypothalamic control of energy expenditure and thermogenesis. Exp Mol Med. 2022;54:358–69. https://doi.org/10.1038/s12276-022-00741-z.
42. Costa-E-sousa RH, Rorato R, Hollenberg AN, Vella KR. Regulation of thyroid hormone levels by hypothalamic thyrotropin-releasing hormone neurons. Thyroid. 2023;33:867–76. https://doi.org/10.1089/thy.2023.0173.
43. Chandrasekar A, Schmidtlein PM, Neve V, Rivagorda M, Spiecker F, Gauthier K, Prevot V, Schwaninger M, Müller-Fielitz H. Regulation of thyroid hormone gatekeepers by thyrotropin in tanycytes. Thyroid. 2024;34:261–73. https://doi.org/10.1089/thy.2023.0375.
44. Milanesi A, Brent GA. Weighing in on thyroid signaling in the hypothalamus: mechanisms and interface with metabolic regulators. Thyroid. 2024;34:141–3. https://doi.org/10.1089/thy.2024.0031.
45. Min SH, Song DK, Lee CH, Roh E, Kim MS. Hypothalamic amp-activated protein kinase as a whole-body energy sensor and regulator. Endocrinol Metab (Seoul). 2024;39:1–11. https://doi.org/10.3803/EnM.2024.1922.
46. Ruska Y, Peterfi Z, Szilvásy-Szabó A, Kővári D, Hrabovszky E, Dorogházi B, Gereben B, Tóth B, Matziari M, Wittmann G, Fekete C. Glp-1 receptor signaling has different effects on the perikarya and axons of the hypophysiotropic thyrotropin-releasing hormone synthesizing neurons in male mice. Thyroid. 2024;34:252–60. https://doi.org/10.1089/thy.2023.0284.
47. Sentis SC, Dore R, Oelkrug R, Kolms B, Iwen KA, Mittag J. Hypothalamic thyroid hormone receptor α1 signaling controls body temperature. Thyroid. 2024;34:243–51. https://doi.org/10.1089/thy.2023.0513.
48. Stepien BK, Huttner WB. Transport, metabolism, and function of thyroid hormones in the developing mammalian brain. Front Endocrinol (Lausanne). 2019;10:209. https://doi.org/10.3389/fendo.2019.00209.
49. Salas-Lucia F, Fekete C, Sinkó R, Egri P, Rada K, Ruska Y, Gereben B, Bianco AC. Axonal T3 uptake and transport can trigger thyroid hormone signaling in the brain. elife. 2023;12:e82683. https://doi.org/10.7554/eLife.82683.
50. Rodríguez-Rodríguez A, Lazcano I, Sánchez-Jaramillo E, Uribe RM, Jaimes-Hoy L, Joseph-Bravo P, Charli JL. Tanycytes and the control of thyrotropin-releasing hormone flux into portal capillaries. Front Endocrinol (Lausanne). 2019;10:401. https://doi.org/10.3389/fendo.2019.00401.
51. Bianco AC, Dumitrescu A, Gereben B, Ribeiro MO, Fonseca TL, Fernandes GW, Bocco BMLC. Paradigms of dynamic control of thyroid hormone signaling. Endocr Rev. 2019;40:1000–47. https://doi.org/10.1210/er.2018-00275.
52. Schussler GC. The thyroxine-binding proteins. Thyroid. 2000;10:141–9. https://doi.org/10.1089/thy.2000.10.141.
53. Groeneweg S, Van Geest FS, Peeters RP, Heuer H, Visser WE. Thyroid hormone transporters. Endocr Rev. 2020;41:bnz008. https://doi.org/10.1210/endrev/bnz008.
54. Flamant F, Cheng SY, Hollenberg AN, Moeller LC, Samarut J, Wondisford FE, Yen PM, Refetoff S. Thyroid hormone signaling pathways: time for a more precise nomenclature. Endocrinology. 2017;158:2052–7. https://doi.org/10.1210/en.2017-00250.
55. Piehl S, Hoefig CS, Scanlan TS, Köhrle J. Thyronamines—past, present, and future. Endocr Rev. 2011;32:64–80. https://doi.org/10.1210/er.2009-0040.
56. Martin JV, Sarkar PK. Nongenomic roles of thyroid hormones and their derivatives in adult brain: are these compounds putative neurotransmitters. Front Endocrinol (Lausanne). 2023;14:1210540. https://doi.org/10.3389/fendo.2023.1210540.
57. Cheng S-Y, Leonard JL, Davis PJ. Molecular aspects of thyroid hormone actions. Endocr Rev. 2010;31:139–70. https://doi.org/10.1210/er.2009-0007.
58. Kahaly GJ, Dillmann WH. Thyroid hormone action in the heart. Endocr Rev. 2005;26:704–28.

59. Korem Kohanim Y, Milo T, Raz M, Karin O, Bar A, Mayo A, Mendelson Cohen N, Toledano Y, Alon U. Dynamics of thyroid diseases and thyroid-axis gland masses. Mol Syst Biol. 2022;18:e10919. https://doi.org/10.15252/msb.202210919.
60. Jaber MA, Benabdelkamel H, Dahabiyeh LA, Masood A, Almalki RH, Musambil M, Alfadda AA, Abdel Rahman AM. The metabolomics approach revealed a distinctive metabolomics pattern associated with hyperthyroidism treatment. Front Endocrinol (Lausanne). 2022;13:1050201. https://doi.org/10.3389/fendo.2022.1050201.
61. Pilo A, Iervasi G, Vitek F, Ferdeghini M, Cazzuola F, Bianchi R. Thyroidal and peripheral production of 3,5,3′-triiodothyronine in humans by multicompartmental analysis. Am J Phys. 1990;258:E715–26. https://doi.org/10.1152/ajpendo.1990.258.4.E715.
62. Bianco AC, Salvatore D, Gereben B, Berry MJ, Larsen PR. Biochemistry, cellular and molecular biology, and physiological roles of the iodothyronine selenodeiodinases. Endocr Rev. 2002;23:38–89. https://doi.org/10.1210/edrv.23.1.0455.
63. Hoermann R, Midgley JEM, Larisch R, Dietrich JW. Integration of peripheral and glandular regulation of triiodothyronine production by thyrotropin in untreated and thyroxine-treated subjects. Horm Metab Res. 2015;47:674–80. https://doi.org/10.1055/s-0034-1398616.
64. Hoermann R, Pekker MJ, Midgley JEM, Larisch R, Dietrich JW. Triiodothyronine secretion in early thyroid failure: the adaptive response of central feedforward control. Eur J Clin Investig. 2020;50:e13192. https://doi.org/10.1111/eci.13192.
65. Ishii H, Inada M, Tanaka K, Mashio Y, Naito K, Nishikawa M, Matsuzuka F, Kuma K, Imura H. Induction of outer and inner ring monodeiodinases in human thyroid gland by thyrotropin. The J Clin Endocrinol Metab. 1983;57:500–5. https://doi.org/10.1210/jcem-57-3-500.
66. Toyoda N, Nishikawa M, Mori Y, Gondou A, Ogawa Y, Yonemoto T, Yoshimura M, Masaki H, Inada M. Thyrotropin and triiodothyronine regulate iodothyronine 5′-deiodinase messenger ribonucleic acid levels in FRTL-5 rat thyroid cells. Endocrinology. 1992;131:389–94. https://doi.org/10.1210/endo.131.1.1319323.
67. Beech SG, Walker SW, Arthur JR, Lee D, Beckett GJ. Differential control of type-i iodothyronine deiodinase expression by the activation of the cyclic amp and phosphoinositol signaling pathways in cultured human thyrocytes. J Mol Endocrinol. 1995;14:171–7. https://doi.org/10.1677/jme.0.0140171.
68. Koenig RJ. Regulation of type 1 iodothyronine deiodinase in health and disease. Thyroid. 2005;15:835–40. https://doi.org/10.1089/thy.2005.15.835.
69. Berberich J, Dietrich JW, Hoermann R, Müller MA. Mathematical modeling of the pituitary-thyroid feedback loop: role of a TSH-t3-shunt and sensitivity analysis. Front Endocrinol (Lausanne). 2018;9:91. https://doi.org/10.3389/fendo.2018.00091.
70. Hoermann R, Pekker MJ, Midgley JEM, Dietrich JW. The role of supporting and disruptive mechanisms of FT3 homeostasis in regulating the hypothalamic-pituitary-thyroid axis. Ther Adv Endocrinol Metab. 2023;14:20420188231158163. https://doi.org/10.1177/20420188231158163.
71. Silvestri E, Schiavo L, Lombardi A, Goglia F. Thyroid hormones as molecular determinants of thermogenesis. Acta Physiol Scand. 2005;184:265–83. https://doi.org/10.1111/j.1365-201X.2005.01463.x.
72. Senese R, Cioffi F, De Lange P, Goglia F, Lanni A. Thyroid: biological actions of "nonclassical" thyroid hormones. J Endocrinol. 2014;221:R1–12. https://doi.org/10.1530/JOE-13-0573.
73. Hoefig CS, Zucchi R, Köhrle J. Thyronamines and derivatives: physiological relevance, pharmacological actions, and future research directions. Thyroid. 2016;26:1656–73. https://doi.org/10.1089/thy.2016.0178.
74. Dietrich JW, Landgrafe G, Fotiadou EH. TSH and thyrotropic agonists: key actors in thyroid homeostasis. J Thyroid Res. 2012;2012:351864. https://doi.org/10.1155/2012/351864.
75. Goede SL, Leow MKS, Smit JW, Klein HH, Dietrich JW. Hypothalamus-pituitary-thyroid feedback control: implications of mathematical modeling and consequences for thyrotropin (tsh) and free thyroxine (ft4) reference ranges. Bull Math Biol. 2014;76:1270–87. https://doi.org/10.1007/s11538-014-9955-5.

76. Hoermann R, Midgley JEM, Larisch R, Dietrich JW. Advances in applied homeostatic modelling of the relationship between thyrotropin and free thyroxine. PLoS One. 2017;12:e0187232. https://doi.org/10.1371/journal.pone.0187232.
77. Danziger L, Elmergreen GL. The thyroid-pituitary homeostatic mechanism. Bull Math Biophys. 1956;18:1–13. https://doi.org/10.1007/BF02477840.
78. Roston S. Mathematical representation of some endocrinological systems. Bull Math Biophys. 1959;21:271–82. https://doi.org/10.1007/BF02477915.
79. Distefano Iii JJ, Stear EB. Neuroendocrine control of thyroid secretion in living systems: a feedback control system model. Bull Math Biophys. 1968;30:3–26. https://doi.org/10.1007/BF02476936.
80. Larsen PR, Silva JE, Kaplan MM. Relationships between circulating and intracellular thyroid hormones: physiological and clinical implications. Endocr Rev. 1981;2:87–102.
81. Dietrich JW. Der Hypophysen-Schilddrüsen-Regelkreis. Berlin: Logos Verlag; 2002. p. 1–188.
82. Dietrich JW, Tesche A, Pickardt CR, Mitzdorf U. Thyrotropic feedback control: evidence for an additional ultrashort feedback loop from fractal analysis. Cybern Syst. 2004;35:315–31. https://doi.org/10.1080/01969720490443354.
83. Spencer CA, Lopresti JS, Patel A, Guttler RB, Eigen A, Shen D, Gray D, Nicoloff JT. Applications of a new chemiluminometric thyrotropin assay to subnormal measurement. J Clin Endocrinol Metab. 1990;70:453–60. https://doi.org/10.1210/jcem-70-2-453.
84. Van Deventer HE, Mendu DR, Remaley AT, Soldin SJ. Inverse log-linear relationship between thyroid-stimulating hormone and free thyroxine measured by direct analog immunoassay and tandem mass spectrometry. Clin Chem. 2011;57:122–7. https://doi.org/10.1373/clinchem.2010.154088.
85. Leow MKS, Goede SL. The homeostatic set point of the hypothalamus-pituitary-thyroid axis—maximum curvature theory for personalized euthyroid targets. Theor Biol Med Model. 2014;11:35. https://doi.org/10.1186/1742-4682-11-35.
86. Goede SL, Leow MKS, Smit JW, Dietrich JW. A novel minimal mathematical model of the hypothalamus-pituitary-thyroid axis validated for individualized clinical applications. Math Biosci. 2014;249:1–7. https://doi.org/10.1016/j.mbs.2014.01.001.
87. Hoermann R, Midgley JEM, Larisch R, Dietrich JW. Relational stability of thyroid hormones in euthyroid subjects and patients with autoimmune thyroid disease. Eur Thyroid J. 2016;5:171–9. https://doi.org/10.1159/000447967.
88. Peeters RP, Brito JP. Subclinical hypothyroidism: to treat or not to treat. Eur J Endocrinol. 2020;183:D15–24. https://doi.org/10.1530/EJE-20-0621.
89. Hoermann R, Midgley JEM, Larisch R, Dietrich JW. Treatment options for subclinical hypothyroidism. Eur J Endocrinol. 2021;185:L5–6. https://doi.org/10.1530/EJE-20-1405.
90. Dietrich JW, Landgrafe-Mende G, Wiora E, Chatzitomaris A, Klein HH, Midgley JEM, Hoermann R. Calculated parameters of thyroid homeostasis: emerging tools for differential diagnosis and clinical research. Front Endocrinol (Lausanne). 2016;7:57. https://doi.org/10.3389/fendo.2016.00057.
91. Andersen S, Pedersen KM, Bruun NH, Laurberg P. Narrow individual variations in serum T4 and T3 in normal subjects: a clue to the understanding of subclinical thyroid disease. J Clin Endocrinol Metab. 2002;87:1068–72. https://doi.org/10.1210/jcem.87.3.8165.
92. Hoermann R, Midgley JEM, Larisch R, Dietrich JW. Individualised requirements for optimum treatment of hypothyroidism: complex needs, limited options. Drugs Context. 2019;8:212597. https://doi.org/10.7573/dic.212597.
93. Gullo D, Latina A, Frasca F, Le Moli R, Pellegriti G, Vigneri R. Levothyroxine monotherapy cannot guarantee euthyroidism in all athyreotic patients. PLoS One. 2011;6:e22552. https://doi.org/10.1371/journal.pone.0022552.
94. Peterson SJ, Cappola AR, Castro MR, Dayan CM, Farwell AP, Hennessey JV, Kopp PA, Ross DS, Samuels MH, Sawka AM, Taylor PN, Jonklaas J, Bianco AC. An online survey of hypo-

thyroid patients demonstrates prominent dissatisfaction. Thyroid. 2018;28:707–21. https://doi.org/10.1089/thy.2017.0681.
95. Pompa M, De Gaetano A, Borri A, Farsetti A, Nanni S, Pontecorvi A, Panunzi S. A physiological mathematical model of the human thyroid. J Comput Sci. 2024;76:102236.
96. Hart Y, Antebi YE, Mayo AE, Friedman N, Alon U. Design principles of cell circuits with paradoxical components. Proc Natl Acad Sci USA. 2012;109:8346–51. https://doi.org/10.1073/pnas.1117475109.
97. Dietrich JW, Hoermann R, Midgley JEM, Bergen F, Müller P. The two faces of Janus: why thyrotropin as a cardiovascular risk factor may be an ambiguous target. Front Endocrinol (Lausanne). 2020;11:829. https://doi.org/10.3389/fendo.2020.542710.
98. Tendler A, Bar A, Mendelsohn-Cohen N, Karin O, Korem Kohanim Y, Maimon L, Milo T, Raz M, Mayo A, Tanay A, Alon U. Hormone seasonality in medical records suggests circannual endocrine circuits. Proc Natl Acad Sci USA. 2021;118(7):e2003926118. https://doi.org/10.1073/pnas.2003926118.
99. Yamada S, Horiguchi K, Akuzawa M, Sakamaki K, Shimomura Y, Kobayashi I, Andou Y, Yamada M. Seasonal variation in thyroid function in over 7,000 healthy subjects in an iodine-sufficient area and literature review. J Endocr Soc. 2022;6:bvac054. https://doi.org/10.1210/jendso/bvac054.
100. Nakao N, Ono H, Yamamura T, Anraku T, Takagi T, Higashi K, Yasuo S, Katou Y, Kageyama S, Uno Y, Kasukawa T, Iigo M, Sharp PJ, Iwasawa A, Suzuki Y, Sugano S, Niimi T, Mizutani M, Namikawa T, Ebihara S, Ueda HR, Yoshimura T. Thyrotrophin in the pars tuberalis triggers photoperiodic response. Nature. 2008;452:317–22. https://doi.org/10.1038/nature06738.
101. Ertek S. Molecular economy of nature with two thyrotropins from different parts of the pituitary: pars tuberalis thyroid-stimulating hormone and pars distalis thyroid-stimulating hormone. Arch Med Sci. 2021;17:189–95. https://doi.org/10.5114/aoms/102476.
102. Gullo D, Latina A, Frasca F, Squatrito S, Belfiore A, Vigneri R. Seasonal variations in TSH serum levels in athyreotic patients under L-thyroxine replacement monotherapy. Clin Endocrinol. 2017;87:207–15. https://doi.org/10.1111/cen.13351.
103. Brabant G, Prank K, Ranft U, Schuermeyer T, Wagner TO, Hauser H, Kummer B, Feistner H, Hesch RD, Von Zur Mühlen A. Physiological regulation of circadian and pulsatile thyrotropin secretion in normal man and woman. J Clin Endocrinol Metab. 1990;70:403–9. https://doi.org/10.1210/jcem-70-2-403.
104. Roelfsema F, Boelen A, Kalsbeek A, Fliers E. Regulatory aspects of the human hypothalamus-pituitary-thyroid axis. Best Pract Res Clin Endocrinol Metab. 2017;31:487–503. https://doi.org/10.1016/j.beem.2017.09.004.
105. Samuels MH, Veldhuis JD, Henry P, Ridgway EC. Pathophysiology of pulsatile and copulsatile release of thyroid-stimulating hormone, luteinizing hormone, follicle-stimulating hormone, and alpha-subunit. J Clin Endocrinol Metab. 1990;71:425–32. https://doi.org/10.1210/jcem-71-2-425.
106. Persani L, Terzolo M, Asteria C, Orlandi F, Angeli A, Beck-Peccoz P. Circadian variations of thyrotropin bioactivity in normal subjects and patients with primary hypothyroidism. J Clin Endocrinol Metab. 1995;80:2722–8.
107. Russell W, Harrison RF, Smith N, Darzy K, Shalet S, Weetman AP, Ross RJ. Free triiodothyronine has a distinct circadian rhythm that is delayed but parallels thyrotropin levels. J Clin Endocrinol Metab. 2008;93:2300–6. https://doi.org/10.1210/jc.2007-2674.
108. Denereaz N, Lemarchand-Beraud T. Severe but not mild alterations of thyroid function modulate the density of thyroid-stimulating hormone receptors in the rat thyroid gland. Endocrinology. 1995;136:1694–700. https://doi.org/10.1210/endo.136.4.7895680.
109. Ehrenkranz J, Bach PR, Snow GL, Schneider A, Lee JL, Ilstrup S, Bennett ST, Benvenga S. Circadian and circannual rhythms in thyroid hormones: determining the TSH and free T4 reference intervals based upon time of day, age, and sex. Thyroid. 2015;25:954–61. https://doi.org/10.1089/thy.2014.0589.

110. Verburg FA, Mäder U, Grelle I, Visser TJ, Peeters RP, Smit JW, Reiners C. The thyroid axis "setpoints" are significantly altered after long-term suppressive LT4 therapy. Horm Metab Res. 2014;46:794–9. https://doi.org/10.1055/s-0034-1375678.
111. Persani L, Borgato S, Romoli R, Asteria C, Pizzocaro A, Beck-Peccoz P. Changes in the degree of sialylation of carbohydrate chains modify the biological properties of circulating thyrotropin isoforms in various physiological and pathological states. J Clin Endocrinol Metab. 1998;83:2486–92. https://doi.org/10.1210/jcem.83.7.4970.

Chapter 6
Mechanisms of Health and Disease

Rudolf Hoermann and Johannes W. Dietrich

6.1 Adaptation and Allostasis

A system designed solely for the purpose of *perfect FT3 homeostasis* could optimally translate its setting from top to bottom, but it would at the same time be firmly locked in by rigid mechanisms, lacking in flexibility, not recognising the need for adapting to new conditions [1]. Such a system, while well suited for the purpose of *homeostasis*, is rather unsupportive of allostasis and the transition to a new state with altered homeostatic levels when this may be more beneficial. An important goal of the thyroid system in all mammalian species is to *synchronise* transitions in the natural environment and their energetic and metabolic consequences [2]. These aspects seem to be particularly important in non-thyroidal diseases [3], but they may be equally relevant for persistent *low-T3 states* that are observed in hypothyroid patients treated with levothyroxine [4]. Therefore, the system of hypothalamic–pituitary–thyroid axis regulation requires additional mechanisms of *homeostatic*

R. Hoermann (✉)
Yandina, QLD, Australia

Department of General Internal Medicine, Gastroenterology and Endocrinology, [Retired] Klinikum Lüdenscheid, Lüdenscheid, Germany
e-mail: rudolf.hoermann@gmail.com

J. W. Dietrich
Diabetes, Endocrinology and Metabolism Section, Department of Medicine, St. Josef-Hospital, Ruhr University Hospitals, Bochum, Germany

Centre for Diabetes Technology (ZDT), Catholic Hospitals Bochum, Bochum, Germany

Centre for Rare Endocrine Diseases (ZSEK), Ruhr Center for Rare Diseases (CeSER), Ruhr University of Bochum and Witten/Herdecke University, Bochum, Germany

Centre for Thyroid Medicine (ZSM), Ruhr University of Bochum, Bochum, Germany
e-mail: johannes.dietrich@ruhr-uni-bochum.de

R. Hoermann, J. W. Dietrich (eds.), *Hypothyroidism*,
https://doi.org/10.1007/978-981-96-3682-2_6

escape and allostatic adaption [1]. A mathematical framework and operational definitions are given in Chap. 4.

This includes aspects of *adaptation* within the organism to meet the diverse energetic and metabolic needs of various organs [1]. To this end, suitable mechanisms are provided by the existence of different sources of T3 generation and their spatio-temporal separation. A degree of *local control* by the tissues, depending on TSH-independent peripheral enzymatic T4 to T3 conversion, supports this goal. The decentralised process generates *extra-thyroidal FT3*, introducing an additional source of T3 directly at the level of each organ, for their own use, but also subject to efflux in the circulation and *in equilibrium* with the circulating FT3 pool. Nevertheless, a strong interconnection with the central system is maintained as

1. The reaction depends on the availability of the *precursor* T4, being, in turn, dependent on appropriate TSH stimulation.
2. Extra-thyroidal FT3 production *feeds back* as a sum effect to the pituitary and hypothalamus to inform the regulatory central organs about the energetic state of the peripheral organs.

   The notion that circulating FT3 signalling to the pituitary informs about the thyroid state of the peripheral organs is consistent with physiological findings that serum and tissue T3 levels are in equilibrium, and the former accurately predict tissue T3 content in peripheral tissues in healthy subjects and patients with hypothyroidism, hyperthyroidism or the non-thyroidal illness (NTI) syndrome [5].

This constitutes an important mechanism of *bottom–up regulation*. On the other hand, *top–down* regulation by TRH and TSH is instrumental in raising the circulating FT4 and FT3 concentrations sufficiently from an otherwise hypothyroid basal state to their healthy euthyroid levels and also adapt the levels precisely as needed in different situations.

We note that the amount contributed by non-thyroidal peripheral FT3 production *varies* by species and also by condition. As mentioned, FT3 efflux from tissues has been estimated to be larger in humans, compared to rodents. *Direct T3 secretion* from the human thyroid gland, while low under normal conditions [6], remains available as a strong rescue mechanism [7]. By opening up *multiple pathways* in support of FT3 production, the system attains a strong and flexible potential of *redundancy* to variably combine different mechanisms [8]. This supports its adaptivity in different physiological conditions to both homeostatic and various allostatic challenges.

Physiologically and clinically, two distinct *phenotypes of thyroid allostasis* can be discerned: type 1 and type 2 allostasis [3] (Table 6.1).

Conditions of *severe illness* and deprivation of energy represent examples of *type 1 allostasis*. Importantly, both the working point of the system and peripheral transfer parameters are altered in these conditions (Table 5.1, Fig. 6.1). In psychosocial stress, pregnancy, metabolic syndrome and adaptation to cold, *type 2 allostasis* is operative, producing a phenotype of predictive *plasticity*. Adaptive responses of thyroid homeostasis explain alterations in thyroid hormone concentrations during

Table 6.1 Types of thyroid allostasis

Type 1 allostasis	Type 2 allostasis
Conditions	*Conditions*
Caloric restriction	Adaption to cold
Exhaustive exercise	Endurance training
Severe illness	Obesity
Depression	Pregnancy
	Post-traumatic stress syndrome
	Schizophrenia
	Bipolar disorders
Hormonal pattern—Acute phase	*Hormonal pattern—Acute phase*
FT3 down	FT3 up
FT4 no change	FT4 no change
TSH no change	TSH up or no change
rT3 up	rT3 down or no change
Hormonal pattern—Chronic phase	*Hormonal pattern—Chronic phase*
FT3 down	FT3 up
FT4 down	FT4 up
TSH down	TSH up
rT3 no change	rT3 up

foetal life, periods of weight gain or weight loss, thermoregulation, physical exercise and psychiatric diseases (Table 6.1, Fig. 6.1). The regulation of the thyroid system is part of a greater system controlling energy metabolism, body weight, fatness and body composition [9–16]. In an attempt to explain obesity, competing theoretical models have been proposed to describe different observable phenomena, but a unifying theoretical model is still lacking [17].

The influence of allostatic factors shifts the location of the achieved observable equilibria between TSH and thyroid hormones in an individual at a time, i.e. the *working point* of the hypothalamic–pituitary–thyroid axis, as illustrated in Fig. 6.1.

6.2 Role of Extra-Thyroidal TSH Receptors

The thyroid is not the only organ expressing a fully *functional TSH receptor* on the cell surface [19]. Other tissues include brown adipose tissue, bone and heart [20–23]. This allows for *bidirectional* communication and additional regulatory circuits linking bottom–up and top–down regulation in the hypothalamic–pituitary–thyroid axis [12, 14, 24]. For instance, adaptation of the working point of the hypothalamic–pituitary–thyroid axis (Fig. 6.1) via *leptin,* a hormone produced by fat cells, links the fat and energy reserves of the body with the central control system, which, in turn, uses the TSH feed-forward to adjust *energy storage and expenditure* [15, 16]. This is a relevant mechanism of type 2 allostasis in obesity [3]. In other examples, TSH inhibits the *RANKL pathway* of osteoclast formation and activation in bone [22]. It antagonises *beta-adrenergic* stimulation in the myocardium and decelerates the physiological rhythm generator in the heart [25].

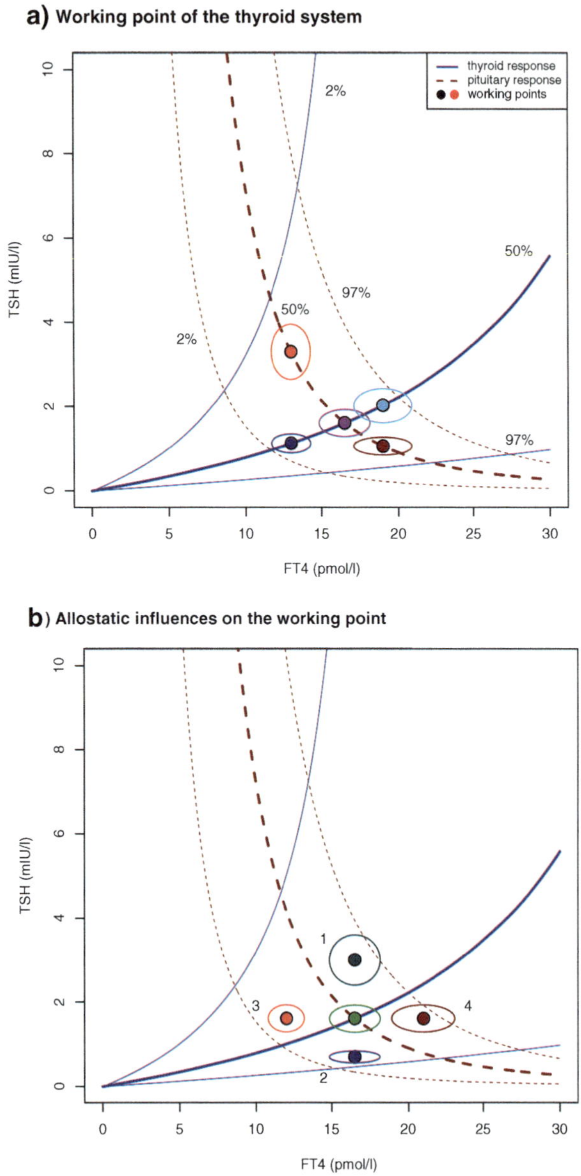

Fig. 6.1 Homeostatic and allostatic challenges to hypothalamic–pituitary–thyroid axis regulation (**a**) Together the thyroid response to TSH (FT4 curve) and the feedback of thyroid hormones on pituitary TSH (TSH curve) define a working point, i.e. the finite equilibrium solution of interlocking TSH–FT4 pairs. Working points are unique to an individual, show little variation, unless disturbed by internal or external strain, and translocate along isoclines. (**b**) Allostatic influences such as obesity, age pregnancy, and non-thyroidal illness have dislocating effects on isoclines and working points [18]. Open circles indicate expected variation (10% for FT4 and 30% for TSH) surrounding a working point characteristic for a person. The area included between the 2.5 and 97.5 percentiles represents the population reference range

6.3 Non-Thyroidal Illness Syndrome

In severely ill hospitalised patients, the *non-thyroidal illness syndrome (NTI)* or *thyroid allostasis in critical illness, tumours, uraemia and starvation* (TACITUS) is commonly observed [26]. Total and free thyroid hormone concentrations are low, FT3 more often so than FT4, and TSH concentrations vary from decreased in severe cases to normal or even elevated in the recovery phase. An acute and chronic phase (wasting syndrome) of TACITUS can be discerned, which differ in mechanisms and prognosis. The acute phase of the allostatic adaption may prove beneficial to the organism, but its persistence in chronic illness leads to allostatic overload, associated with poor outcome. For clinicians, the various forms of thyroid allostasis pose serious problems in the *differential diagnosis* of thyroid diseases [3].

An older term synonymous to the non-thyroid illness syndrome is the *low-T3 syndrome*. However, low FT3 concentrations observed in the context of type 1 allostatic load, non-thyroidal illness or TACITUS syndrome are generally not regarded as a form of hypothyroidism, rather as a temporary adaptive energy-saving response to any severe disease. Interactions with the stress response of the hypothalamic–pituitary–adrenal axis occur [27]. The observed thyroid hormone pattern and low T3 concentrations cannot be explained by changes in peripheral deiodinase activity alone [3]. Rather multiple homeostatic mechanisms are altered, leading to the synchronisation of central and peripheral mechanisms in the *disruption* of the normal hypothalamic–pituitary–thyroid axis regulation. The low-T3 syndrome arises from a combination of peripheral hypodeiodination and central hyperdeiodination, a seeming paradox explained by spatial diversity and feedback effects [3] (Fig. 6.2). While peripheral FT3 concentrations rise due to increasing sum activity of peripheral type 1 deiodinase, central FT3 concentrations decrease with increasing type 2 deiodinase activity. Consequently, increased central T3 signalling suppresses the release of TRH and TSH. Change is mainly induced by lipopolysaccharide, cytokines, such as IL-12 and IL-8 and, possibly, increased concentrations of 3,5-diiodothyronine, triiodothyroacetate and tetra-iodothyroacetate during the acute phase response. The scenario is predicted by mathematical modelling and agrees with experimental studies in animals in vivo [3, 26, 28–32].

Type 3 deiodinase is upregulated in TACITUS, increasing the production and serum concentrations of rT3, which may, in turn, inhibit thyroid hormone

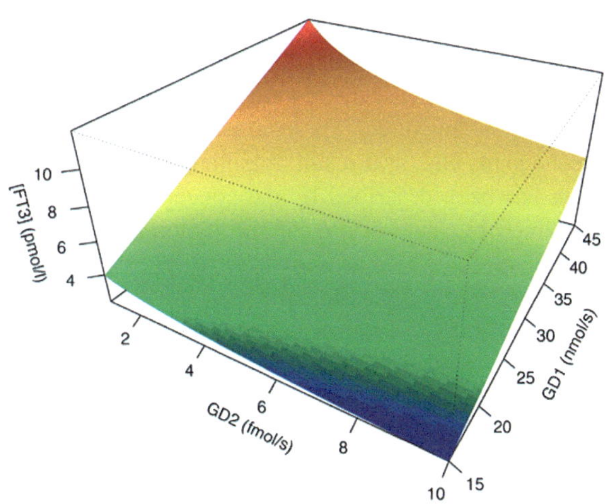

Fig. 6.2 Combination of peripheral and central mechanisms leading to the low-T3 syndrome
The activities of peripheral (GD1) and central (GD2) deiodinases diverge to cause the low-T3 phenotype [34]. See text for details. (The graph shown has been produced by computer simulation with the free app SimThyr [33])

signalling. Apart from the main mechanisms disruptive to normal hypothalamic–pituitary–thyroid regulation described here, a multitude of metabolic changes and affected physiological pathways exists in critical illness, summarised elsewhere [3].

Clinically, depending on the severity of the disease, the low-T3 syndrome may be accompanied by low FT4 concentrations and low, normal or moderately elevated (recovery phase) TSH concentrations [34]. Diagnostically, these hormonal changes must always be interpreted in a clinical context and with the full knowledge of the history and symptoms of the patient.

Treatment of the non-thyroid illness syndrome with thyroid hormones is generally not recommended [3]. Whether or not thyroid hormone replacement may be beneficial to some patients with the condition, particularly when persistent, is controversial.

A shared phenomenon across the diverse spectrum of allostatic responses is that homeostatic mechanisms are disrupted, asymmetric movements arise and the equilibria (balance) between the interacting hormones are shifted [7]. The resulting changes may be unexpected and are difficult to predict, given the interdependent nature of thyroid parameters, acting as controlling and controlled variables, and their asymmetric non-linear behaviour. They are frequently incompatible with basic assumptions of conventional statistical tests, requiring more advanced statistical analysis or a mathematical modelling approach to be fully appreciated.

6.4 Early Thyroid Failure and Subclinical Hypothyroidism

Disruptive mechanisms of homeostasis lead to disease [35]. Autoimmune thyroiditis is a chronic disease destroying functional thyroid tissue in the process of its slow progression. The destructive process thereby results in a slowly progressive *decline of thyroid hormone production* by the thyroid, presenting a challenge of capacity stress to the hypothalamic–pituitary–thyroid axis regulation [36]. As T4 production and release decline, FT4 concentration also decreases, resulting in a pituitary response of releasing more TSH. The increase in pituitary TSH activates the TSH-T3 shunt, i.e. TSH feed-forward on T4 to T3 conversion [36–38]. It also increases TSH-dependent direct T3 secretion [8]. FT3 homeostasis is supported by these mechanisms and, as a result, maintained in early thyroid failure [4]. This phenomenon has been described by the concept of *relational stability* (see Chap. 2) and explained by the working of the hypothalamic–pituitary–thyroid axis regulation (see Chap. 5).

As a clinical implication, the laboratory constellation of *subclinical hypothyroidism* in early thyroid failure cannot routinely be regarded as a hypothyroid diseased state. Rather the corrective actions of TSH appear to be able to maintain in a state of relational stability the normal functioning of thyroid-hormone dependent processes (Fig. 6.3). This is particularly true for the T3-dependent genomic actions, at least in early thyroid failure. Clinical studies support the model predictions in this respect [36]. Consequently, early levothyroxine substitution should be withheld in these patients, particularly if they are asymptomatic, as the administration of the exogenous hormone suppresses TSH, thereby further weakening the support for FT3 homeostasis and potentially decreasing circulating FT3 concentrations.

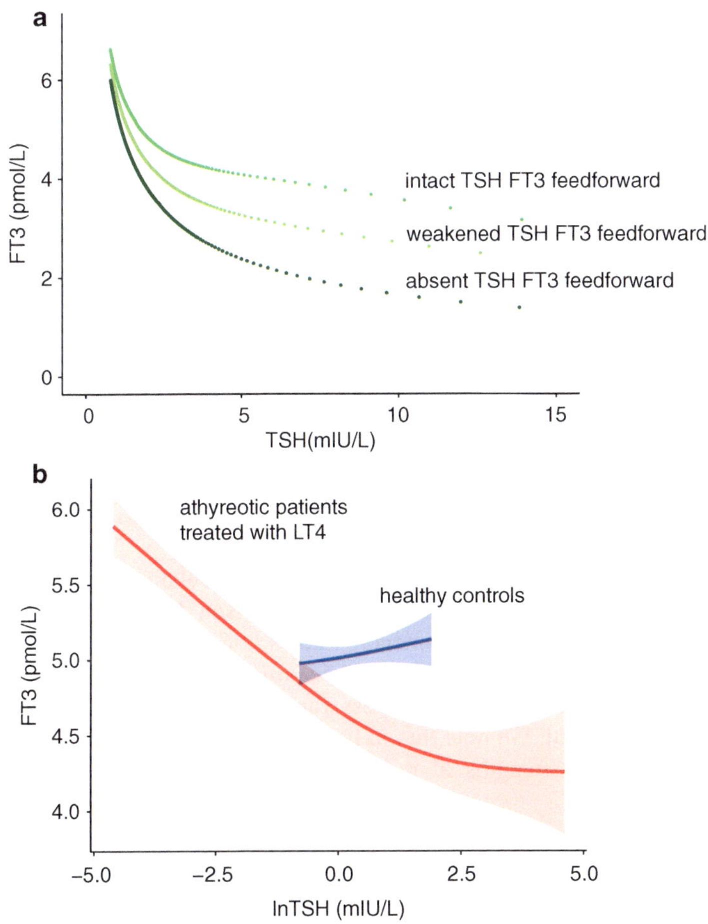

Fig. 6.3 Loss of FT3 homeostasis
(**a**) Theoretical modelling predicts a loss of FT3 homeostasis if the TSH feed-forward on FT3 is weakened or absent. (Modified according to Hoermann et al. [7]). (**b**) This agrees with the loss of relational stability and FT3 homeostasis observed in athyreotic patients with thyroid carcinoma on LT4 replacement. Regression lines with 95% confidence intervals (shaded area) shown here were fitted with general additive models. While FT3 levels were uncorrelated to logarithmic TSH in the healthy controls (n = 207), FT3 became homeostatically unstable in the patients (n = 353). (Modified from Hoermann et al. [4], based on data from Hoermann et al. [39])

6.5 Thyroid Failure and Hypothyroidism

When the thyroid volume and/or its functional capacity become too low in progressive autoimmune thyroiditis or for other reasons such as thyroidectomy, *primary hypothyroidism* ensues. In this condition, both FT4 concentrations decrease below normal and FT3 homeostasis can no longer be maintain by the system at its previous level. The supporting mechanisms of FT3 homeostasis are *broken* due to both a lack of substrate and the loss of sufficient intact thyroid tissue expressing TSH-dependent T4 to T3 converting enzymes and/or secreting T3 [7, 8] (Fig. 6.3).

The *loss of the physiological TSH feed-forward* on FT3 profoundly alters the resulting equilibria and balance between the three hormones TSH, FT4 and FT3. The previously "normal" level of TSH is now associated with a relative "low-T3 syndrome" on levothyroxine replacement, as the system finds a new equilibrium with increased FT4 concentrations and decreased TSH and FT3 concentrations [4, 18, 40]. To restore the previous "normal" FT3 level under these conditions, it is often necessary to raise FT4 concentrations substantially and beyond the upper limit of its reference range, thereby suppressing TSH concentration below reference [41]. It follows that the absolute TSH level cannot be regarded as a reliable indicator of euthyroidism. Nor is a suppressed TSH alone under these circumstances indicative of the presence of a thyrotoxic state, because its association with a relatively low FT3 level describes a situation entirely different from endogenous hyperthyroidism where the suppressed TSH combines with an increased FT3 concentration [42]. In LT4-treated athyreotic patents, the probability of raising FT3 concentrations above midrange remains lower than the probability of suppressing TSH levels below the lower reference limit [43].

These findings relate to FT3 homeostasis in the circulation. T3 homeostasis in human tissues is not readily explorable for comparison due to the invasive nature of such studies. However, experimental studies conducted in tissues of rodents agree with these findings, demonstrating the *inability of levothyroxine replacement alone* to restore normal T3 levels across various tissues despite achieving TSH normalisation [44–46]. We note that in humans and rodents qualitative responses are similar but the strengths of the different T3-generating pathways are not the same.

In healthy controls, serum FT3 concentrations are *uncorrelated* with logarithmic TSH levels while being maintained at a homeostatic level by the opposing actions of TSH and FT4. Thereby, supporting actions of TSH on FT3 display a strong *relational stability* (see Chap. 2). However, in athyreotic patients on LT4 replacement, *disruptive mechanisms* cause a loss of the former relational stability between the hormones (Fig. 6.3). In these patients, the homeostatic level of FT3 is no longer preserved, and FT3 levels are now proportionally *correlated* with T4 supply and TSH concentrations (Fig. 6.3). *Broken FT3 homeostasis* leads to an unstable system. The implications and predicted consequences of these findings for patient care are profound. They will be discussed later.

6.6 Reduced Sensitivity to Thyroid Hormone

The observation of high thyroid hormone levels in some patients in the absence of any apparent signs or symptoms of hypothyroidism or hyperthyroidism and a lack of TSH suppression led to the discovery of the *syndrome of resistance to thyroid hormone* (RTH) [47]. A common form of the variable clinical syndrome has been identified as a hereditary disease caused by mutations in the thyroid hormone receptor beta (*THRB*) gene, termed *RTHβ* [48]. Although most individuals with the syndrome are considered clinically euthyroid, this is not invariably true. In some patients, *THRB mutations* may be differentially expressed by tissue types, rendering organs selectively hyperthyroid or hypothyroid at the level of the tissue response in the same individual. The terms generalised RTH, isolated pituitary RTH and peripheral tissue RTH describe different clinical manifestations of RTHβ, with generalised RTH being the most prevalent and euthyroid manifestation of the syndrome. No specific therapy is currently available to fully correct the *THRβ* defect. Treatment with levothyroxine is mainly aimed at preventing the growth-promoting effect of elevated TSH levels and consecutive goitre formation. *TRα gene defects* (also known as *THRA*) have long been suspected to exist but were only identified as a cause of the clinically variable RTH syndrome decades later [49]. The clinical presentation of patients is diverse, but normocytic or macrocytic anaemia may be a common feature of that syndrome [50].

With the discovery of more defects in the extra- and intra-cellular pathway of thyroid hormone action, such as in the transmembrane transport of thyroid hormones (for instance caused by *MCT8* mutations) a new term was coined, namely *reduced sensitivity to thyroid hormone* [47].

While the differentiation and differential treatment of the various forms of the RTH syndrome have become a rapidly emerging perplex field and require a highly specialised area of expertise, a reduced sensitivity to thyroid hormone is shared among the syndromes. This hallmark of the disease, namely a *non-suppressed TSH despite an increase in thyroid hormone levels* should raise clinical suspicion and prompt further investigation. These syndromes of reduced, but compensated sensitivity to thyroid hormones must not be confused with the far more prevalent disease of primary hypothyroidism, where the TSH level is elevated in association with reduced circulating FT4 concentrations.

In some cases, the resistance to thyroid hormone does not equally affect both thyroid hormones (T4 and T3) but is specific to T4. These patients show a *reduced T4-sensitivity* to downregulate TSH, but normal T3-sensitivity to TSH downregulation [51]. They are characterised by a lack of TSH suppression in response to LT4 treatment, despite achieving high circulating FT4 concentrations, together with a low FT3 to FT4 ratio and low circulating FT3 concentrations. The disease mechanism is unknown, but a post-translational defect in the deiodinase type 2 pathway has been suspected [51]. Treatment of these patients should include T3 substitution.

6.6.1 Acquired Syndromes of Resistance to Thyroid Hormone

Another hypothyroid disorder, distinguishable from both primary hypothyroidism and compensated resistance syndromes to thyroid hormones, is the constellation of a patient presenting with the typical spectrum of symptoms and clinical manifestation of hypothyroidism, yet seemingly unremarkable results of thyroid function testing that, contrary to the clinical presentation, suggest the presence of biochemical euthyroidism. This type of hypothyroidism typically belongs to the spectrum of *acquired syndromes of resistance to thyroid hormone*. Suspicion arises not so much from the biochemical test results but from the sharp discrepancy between the clinical picture and the laboratory results. The main cause of the variably expressed clinical syndromes from mild to severe forms of true hypothyroidism are the actions of multiple chemical compounds interfering with the functions of the endocrine system at a spectrum of sites including those of thyroid hormones [52–56]. These chemicals include prevalent toxins and pollutants found in the environment in modern society. They have been termed *endocrine disruptors* [57–59]. Because the thyroid system is complex, it presents many potential targets to the disrupting actions of these chemicals in the path of thyroid hormone actions [54]. Different chemicals, including certain pharmacological drugs, can inhibit iodide uptake, decrease thyroid hormone synthesis and circulating levels of thyroid hormones, impair distribution and transport proteins and interfere with thyroid hormone receptor binding. Their actions may also insidiously combine to inflict multi-hit defects to the system and affect various steps of regulation in a combined manner. In particular, the interfering actions at the endpoint of the cellular T3 response, the nuclear DNA-binding sites, explain the expression of a hypothyroid syndrome in the presence of "normal" circulating concentrations of thyroid hormones but unresponsive to them. We note that *summation effects* of multiple prevalent toxins are inadequately addressed by thresholds of toxicological concern for individual substances.

References

1. Hoermann R, Pekker M, Midgley JEM, Larisch R, Dietrich JW. Principles of endocrine regulation: reconciling tensions between robustness in performance and adaptation to change. Front Endocrinol (Lausanne). 2022;13:825107. https://doi.org/10.3389/fendo.2022.825107.
2. Zwahlen J, Gairin E, Vianello S, Mercader M, Roux N, Laudet V. The ecological function of thyroid hormones. Philos Trans R Soc Lond Ser B Biol Sci. 2024;379:20220511. https://doi.org/10.1098/rstb.2022.0511.
3. Chatzitomaris A, Hoermann R, Midgley JEM, Hering S, Urban A, Dietrich B, Abood A, Klein HH, Dietrich JW. Thyroid allostasis-adaptive responses of thyrotropic feedback control to conditions of strain, stress, and developmental programming. Front Endocrinol (Lausanne). 2017;8:163. https://doi.org/10.3389/fendo.2017.00163.
4. Hoermann R, Midgley JEM, Larisch R, Dietrich JW. Relational stability in the expression of normality, variation, and control of thyroid function. Front Endocrinol (Lausanne). 2016;7:142. https://doi.org/10.3389/fendo.2016.00142.

5. Salas-Lucia F, Bianco AC. T3 levels and thyroid hormone signaling. Front Endocrinol (Lausanne). 2022;13:1044691. https://doi.org/10.3389/fendo.2022.1044691.
6. Bianco AC, Dumitrescu A, Gereben B, Ribeiro MO, Fonseca TL, Fernandes GW, Bocco BMLC. Paradigms of dynamic control of thyroid hormone signaling. Endocr Rev. 2019;40:1000–47. https://doi.org/10.1210/er.2018-00275.
7. Hoermann R, Pekker MJ, Midgley JEM, Dietrich JW. The role of supporting and disruptive mechanisms of FT3 homeostasis in regulating the hypothalamic-pituitary-thyroid axis. Ther Adv Endocrinol Metab. 2023;14:20420188231158163. https://doi.org/10.1177/20420188231158163.
8. Hoermann R, Pekker MJ, Midgley JEM, Larisch R, Dietrich JW. Triiodothyronine secretion in early thyroid failure: the adaptive response of central feedforward control. Eur J Clin Investig. 2020;50:e13192. https://doi.org/10.1111/eci.13192.
9. Menendez C, Baldelli R, Camiña JP, Escudero B, Peino R, Dieguez C, Casanueva FF. TSH stimulates leptin secretion by a direct effect on adipocytes. J Endocrinol. 2003;176:7–12. https://doi.org/10.1677/joe.0.1760007.
10. Joseph-Bravo P. Hypophysiotropic thyrotropin-releasing hormone neurons as transducers of energy homeostasis. Endocrinology. 2004;145:4813–5. https://doi.org/10.1210/en.2004-0979.
11. Lechan RM, Fekete C. The TRH neuron: a hypothalamic integrator of energy metabolism. Prog Brain Res. 2006;153:209–35. https://doi.org/10.1016/S0079-6123(06)53012-2.
12. Biondi B. Thyroid and obesity: an intriguing relationship. J Clin Endocrinol Metab. 2010;95:3614–7. https://doi.org/10.1210/jc.2010-1245.
13. Reinehr T. Thyroid function in the nutritionally obese child and adolescent. Curr Opin Pediatr. 2011;23:415–20. https://doi.org/10.1097/MOP.0b013e328344c393.
14. Mullur R, Liu YY, Brent GA. Thyroid hormone regulation of metabolism. Physiol Rev. 2014;94:355–82. https://doi.org/10.1152/physrev.00030.2013.
15. Hoermann R, Cheung AS, Milne M, Grossmann M. Hypothalamic-pituitary-thyroid axis set point alterations are associated with body composition in androgen-deprived men. J Endocr Soc. 2017;1:874–85. https://doi.org/10.1210/js.2017-00057.
16. Liu Z, Xiao T, Liu H. Leptin signaling and its central role in energy homeostasis. Front Neurosci. 2023;17:1238528. https://doi.org/10.3389/fnins.2023.1238528.
17. Speakman JR, Hall KD. Models of body weight and fatness regulation. Philos Trans R Soc B Biol Sci. 2023;378:3. https://doi.org/10.1098/rstb.2022.0231.
18. Hoermann R, Midgley JEM, Larisch R, Dietrich JW. Recent advances in thyroid hormone regulation: toward a new paradigm for optimal diagnosis and treatment. Front Endocrinol (Lausanne). 2017;8:364. https://doi.org/10.3389/fendo.2017.00364.
19. Vassart G, Dumont JE. The thyrotropin receptor and the regulation of thyrocyte function and growth. Endocr Rev. 1992;13:596–611. https://doi.org/10.1210/edrv-13-3-596.
20. De Lloyd A, Bursell J, Gregory JW, Rees DA, Ludgate M. TSH receptor activation and body composition. J Endocrinol. 2010;204:13–20. https://doi.org/10.1677/JOE-09-0262.
21. Williams GR. Extrathyroidal expression of TSH receptor. Ann Endocrinol (Paris). 2011;72:68–73. https://doi.org/10.1016/j.ando.2011.03.006.
22. Fröhlich E, Wahl R. Mechanisms in endocrinology: impact of isolated TSH levels in and out of normal range on different tissues. Eur J Endocrinol. 2016;174:R29–41. https://doi.org/10.1530/EJE-15-0713.
23. Vieira IH, Rodrigues D, Paiva I. The mysterious universe of the TSH receptor. Front Endocrinol (Lausanne). 2022;13:944715. https://doi.org/10.3389/fendo.2022.944715.
24. Pleić N, Gunjača I, Babić Leko M, Zemunik T. Thyroid function and metabolic syndrome: a two-sample bidirectional mendelian randomization study. J Clin Endocrinol Metab. 2023;108:3190–200. https://doi.org/10.1210/clinem/dgad371.
25. Müller P, Leow MK, Dietrich JW. Minor perturbations of thyroid homeostasis and major cardiovascular endpoints-physiological mechanisms and clinical evidence. Front Cardiovasc Med. 2022;9:942971. https://doi.org/10.3389/fcvm.2022.942971.

26. Fliers E, Bianco AC, Langouche L, Boelen A. Thyroid function in critically ill patients. Lancet Diabetes Endocrinol. 2015;3:816–25.
27. Langouche L, Téblick A, Gunst J, Van Den Berghe G. The hypothalamus-pituitary-adrenocortical response to critical illness: a concept in need of revision. Endocr Rev. 2023;44:1096–106. https://doi.org/10.1210/endrev/bnad021.
28. Degroot LJ. "Non-thyroidal illness syndrome" is functional central hypothyroidism, and if severe, hormone replacement is appropriate in light of present knowledge. J Endocrinol Investig. 2003;26:1163–70. https://doi.org/10.1007/BF03349151.
29. Fekete C, Gereben B, Doleschall M, Harney JW, Dora JM, Bianco AC, Sarkar S, Liposits Z, Rand W, Emerson C, Kacskovics I, Larsen PR, Lechan RM. Lipopolysaccharide induces type 2 iodothyronine deiodinase in the mediobasal hypothalamus: implications for the nonthyroidal illness syndrome. Endocrinology. 2004;145:1649–55. https://doi.org/10.1210/en.2003-1439.
30. Lechan RM, Fekete C. Feedback regulation of thyrotropin-releasing hormone (trh): mechanisms for the non-thyroidal illness syndrome. J Clin Endocrinol Metab. 2004;27:105–19.
31. Mebis L, Van Den Berghe G. The hypothalamus-pituitary-thyroid axis in critical illness. Neth J Med. 2009;67:332–40.
32. Wajner SM, Maia AL. New insights toward the acute non-thyroidal illness syndrome. Front Endocrinol (Lausanne). 2012;3:8. https://doi.org/10.3389/fendo.2012.00008.
33. Dietrich JW. Simthyr 4.0.1. https://simthyr.sourceforge.io. rrid: Scr_014351. 2019. https://doi.org/10.5281/zenodo.1303822. Accessed 15 Apr 2024.
34. Van Den Berghe G. Non-thyroidal illness in the ICU: a syndrome with different faces. Thyroid. 2014;24:1456–65. https://doi.org/10.1089/thy.2014.0201.
35. Billman GE. Homeostasis: the underappreciated and far too often ignored central organizing principle of physiology. Front Physiol. 2020;11:200. https://doi.org/10.3389/fphys.2020.00200.
36. Hoermann R, Midgley JEM, Larisch R, Dietrich JW. Relational stability of thyroid hormones in euthyroid subjects and patients with autoimmune thyroid disease. Eur Thyroid J. 2016;5:171–9. https://doi.org/10.1159/000447967.
37. Ishii H, Inada M, Tanaka K, Mashio Y, Naito K, Nishikawa M, Matsuzuka F, Kuma K, Imura H. Induction of outer and inner ring monodeiodinases in human thyroid gland by thyrotropin. J Clin Endocrinol Metab. 1983;57:500–5. https://doi.org/10.1210/jcem-57-3-500.
38. Berberich J, Dietrich JW, Hoermann R, Müller MA. Mathematical modeling of the pituitary-thyroid feedback loop: role of a TSH-t3-shunt and sensitivity analysis. Front Endocrinol (Lausanne). 2018;9:91. https://doi.org/10.3389/fendo.2018.00091.
39. Hoermann R, Midgley JEM, Giacobino A, Eckl WA, Wahl HG, Dietrich JW, Larisch R. Homeostatic equilibria between free thyroid hormones and pituitary thyrotropin are modulated by various influences including age, body mass index and treatment. Clin Endocrinol. 2014;81:907–15. https://doi.org/10.1111/cen.12527.
40. Jansen HI, Bult MM, Bisschop PH, Boelen A, Heijboer AC, Hillebrand JJ. Increased FT4 concentrations in patients using levothyroxine without complete suppression of TSH. Endocr Connect. 2023;12:e220538. https://doi.org/10.1530/EC-22-0538.
41. Hoermann R, Midgley JEM, Larisch R, Dietrich JW. Individualised requirements for optimum treatment of hypothyroidism: complex needs, limited options. Drugs Context. 2019;8:212597. https://doi.org/10.7573/dic.212597.
42. Hoermann R, Midgley JEM, Larisch R, Dietrich JW. Heterogenous biochemical expression of hormone activity in subclinical/overt hyperthyroidism and exogenous thyrotoxicosis. J Clin Trans Endocrinol. 2020;19:100219. https://doi.org/10.1016/j.jcte.2020.100219.
43. Midgley JEM, Larisch R, Dietrich JW, Hoermann R. Variation in the biochemical response to L-thyroxine therapy and relationship with peripheral thyroid hormone conversion efficiency. Endocr Connect. 2015;4:196–205. https://doi.org/10.1530/EC-15-0056.
44. Escobar-Morreale HF, Obregón MJ, Escobar Del Rey F, Morereale De Escobar G. Replacement therapy for hypothyroidism with thyroxine alone does not ensure euthyroidism in all tissues, as studied in thyroidectomized rats. J Clin Invest. 1995;96:2828–38. https://doi.org/10.1172/JCI118353.

45. Werneck De Castro JP, Fonseca TL, Ueta CB, Mcaninch EA, Abdalla SM, Wittmann G, Lechan RM, Gereben B, Bianco AC. Differences in hypothalamic type 2 deiodinase ubiquitination explain localized sensitivity to thyroxine. J Clin Invest. 2015;125:769–81. https://doi.org/10.1172/JCI77588.
46. McAninch EA, Bianco AC. New insights into the variable effectiveness of levothyroxine monotherapy for hypothyroidism. Lancet Diabetes Endocrinol. 2015;3:756–8. https://doi.org/10.1016/S2213-8587(15)00325-3.
47. Dumitrescu AM, Refetoff S. The syndromes of reduced sensitivity to thyroid hormone. Biochim Biophys Acta. 2013;1830:3987–4003. https://doi.org/10.1016/j.bbagen.2012.08.005.
48. Grasberger H, Refetoff S. Resistance to thyrotropin. Best Pract Res Clin Endocrinol Metab. 2017;31:183–94. https://doi.org/10.1016/j.beem.2017.03.004.
49. Dahll LK, Westbye AB, Vinorum K, Sejersted Y, Barøy T, Thorsby PM, Hammerstad SS. Clinical and biochemical characteristics of untreated adult patients with resistance to thyroid hormone alpha. J Endocr Soc. 2023;7:bvad089. https://doi.org/10.1210/jendso/bvad089.
50. Kağızmanlı GA, Kırbıyık Ö, Abacı A, Böber E, Yiş U, Demir K. Anaemia-based screening for resistance to thyroid hormone alpha in children. Clin Endocrinol. 2023; https://doi.org/10.1111/cen.15007.
51. Lacámara N, Lecumberri B, Barquiel B, Escribano A, González-Casado I, Álvarez-Escolá C, Aleixandre-Blanquer F, Morales F, Alfayate R, Bernal-Soriano MC, Miralles R, Yildirim Simsir I, Özgen AG, Bernal J, Berbel P, Moreno JC. Identification of resistance to exogenous thyroxine in humans. Thyroid. 2020;30:1732–44. https://doi.org/10.1089/thy.2019.0825.
52. Lauretta R, Sansone A, Sansone M, Romanelli F, Appetecchia M. Endocrine disrupting chemicals: effects on endocrine glands. Front Endocrinol (Lausanne). 2019;10:178. https://doi.org/10.3389/fendo.2019.00178.
53. Graceli JB, Dettogni RS, Merlo E, Niño O, Da Costa CS, Zanol JF, Morris EAR, Miranda-Alves L, Denicol AC. The impact of endocrine-disrupting chemical exposure in the mammalian hypothalamic-pituitary axis. Mol Cell Endocrinol. 2020;518:110997.
54. Homburg M, Rasmussen ÅK, Ramhøj L, Feldt-Rasmussen U. The influence of triclosan on the thyroid hormone system in humans—a systematic review. Front Endocrinol (Lausanne). 2022;13:883827. https://doi.org/10.3389/fendo.2022.883827.
55. Bagga AD, Johnson BP, Zhang Q. A minimal human physiologically based kinetic model of thyroid hormones and chemical disruption of plasma thyroid hormone binding proteins. Front Endocrinol (Lausanne). 2023;14:1168663. https://doi.org/10.3389/fendo.2023.1168663.
56. Forner-Piquer I, Baig AH, Kortenkamp A. Disruption of the thyroid hormone system and patterns of altered thyroid hormones after gestational chemical exposures in rodents—a systematic review. Front Endocrinol (Lausanne). 2024;14:1323284. https://doi.org/10.3389/fendo.2023.1323284.
57. Gore AC, Chappell VA, Fenton SE, Flaws JA, Nadal A, Prins GS, Toppari J, Zoeller RT. Edc-2: the endocrine society's second scientific statement on endocrine-disrupting chemicals. Endocr Rev. 2015;36:E1–E150. https://doi.org/10.1210/er.2015-1010.
58. Schug TT, Johnson AF, Birnbaum LS, Colborn T, Guillette LJ, Crews DP, Collins T, Soto AM, Vom Saal FS, Mclachlan JA, Sonnenschein C, Heindel JJ. Minireview: endocrine disruptors: past lessons and future directions. Mol Endocrinol. 2016;30:833–47. https://doi.org/10.1210/me.2016-1096.
59. Demeneix B, Vandenberg LN, Ivell R, Zoeller RT. Thresholds and endocrine disruptors: an endocrine society policy perspective. J Endocr Soc. 2020;4:bvaa085. https://doi.org/10.1210/jendso/bvaa085.

Chapter 7
Approach to the Patient

Rudolf Hoermann and Johannes W. Dietrich

The *approach to a patient* with suspected hypothyroidism starts with patient symptoms, taking a detailed history and examination of the patient, followed by laboratory evaluation including thyroid function tests, markers of autoimmunity, other hormones and laboratory tests of interest. Ultrasonography of the thyroid routinely complements and augments the clinical examination of the organ.

7.1 Symptoms of Hypothyroidism

The expression of the *symptom spectrum* in hypothyroidism is highly variable, with some patients experiencing few or no apparent symptoms (oligosymptomatic or asymptomatic forms) and others showing more characteristic signs and symptoms of the disease [1]. This heterogeneity of symptoms reflects individual differences in

R. Hoermann (✉)
Yandina, QLD, Australia

Department of General Internal Medicine, Gastroenterology and Endocrinology, [Retired] Klinikum Lüdenscheid, Lüdenscheid, Germany
e-mail: rudolf.hoermann@gmail.com

J. W. Dietrich
Diabetes, Endocrinology and Metabolism Section, Department of Medicine, St. Josef-Hospital, Ruhr University Hospitals, Bochum, Germany

Centre for Diabetes Technology (ZDT), Catholic Hospitals Bochum, Bochum, Germany

Centre for Rare Endocrine Diseases (ZSEK), Ruhr Center for Rare Diseases (CeSER), Ruhr University of Bochum and Witten/Herdecke University, Bochum, Germany

Centre for Thyroid Medicine (ZSM), Ruhr University of Bochum, Bochum, Germany
e-mail: johannes.dietrich@ruhr-uni-bochum.de

R. Hoermann, J. W. Dietrich (eds.), *Hypothyroidism*,
https://doi.org/10.1007/978-981-96-3682-2_7

the sensitivity to thyroid hormones, the central working point of the feedback control system and current context factors, including comorbidity. Typically, hypothyroid symptoms are an expression of an *energy-deficiency syndrome* and the *slowdown* of a multitude of metabolic pathways and bodily functions, which cannot be sustained in the absence of sufficient thyroid hormone supply and effects. The most characteristic symptoms are tiredness, fatigue, loss of energy, physical and mental decline, weakness, intolerance to cold environment, hypothermia, weight gain despite low appetite, bradycardia, hyporeflexia, depressive symptoms, hair loss, constipation, irregularities of the menstrual cycle in women, decline of libido and sexual function in men (Table 7.1).

The experienced doctor may recognise when present the *pathognomic* aspect of a patient presenting with hypothyroidism. *Signs to look for* are a turgid face, eyelid oedema, reduced facial expression, pale and dry skin, coarse and scrubby hair and enlarged tongue. The voice often sounds hoarse, the language is retarded and motor functions are reduced and slow. The body temperature may be lower than average. Cardiac symptoms that may raise suspicion of hypothyroidism in the first place include bradycardia, myocardial insufficiency, pleural effusions and paroxysmal hypertension. Associations between hypothyroidism and alterations in heart rate variability have also been documented, affecting cardiac autonomic function [2].

Hypothyroid myopathy with progressive muscle weakness is another not so well-known sign.

At the onset of the disease, subtle and less specific symptoms prevail, such as fatigue, exhaustion, lack of performance, lack of concentration and mood swings, so that the specific diagnosis is often missed and symptoms are attributed to other causes or the ageing process.

We note that even in the absence of symptoms and hormonal deficiencies immunological markers, particularly thyroid peroxidase (TPO) antibodies, may be early indicators of the underlying disease process.

Clinical examination can recognise the overall hypothyroid impression described above, assess the Achilles tendon reflex, dry cold skin, a slow heartbeat, a hypertensive blood pressure and the morphology of the thyroid gland. *Myxedematous coma*, on the other hand, is an extreme clinical condition of hypothyroidism. The exacerbation is frequently precipitated by other stressful events such as infections. It represents a decompensated life-threatening clinical disease with multiple organ abnormalities that requires intensive care treatment.

7.2 Patient History

Taking the *history of a patient* suspected to suffer from hypothyroidism typically addresses the following questions:

Thyroid diseases or autoimmune disorders in the family
Previous thyroid surgery, radioiodine treatment or radiation in the neck region

Table 7.1 Symptomatic disease spectrum of hypothyroidism

General symptoms
Decreased performance, fatigue, tiredness Weight gain, cold intolerance
Glandular symptoms
Smaller or less frequently enlarged thyroid
Cardiovascular system
Bradycardia Reduced cardiac output, cardiomegaly, pericardial effusion (rare) Arterial hypotension, paradox hypertension Heart rate variability
Pulmonary system
Difficulty breathing, hypercapnia
Skin and skin appendages
Dry and pale skin, hair loss, brittle nails Pretibial myxoedema (rare, more frequent in Graves' disease)
Eye signs
Eyelid oedema Exophthalmos (rare, more frequent in Graves' disease)
Mouth and tongue
Macroglossia Slurred language Deep, hoarse voice
Nervous system
Lack of energy, apathy, sleepiness, poor concentration, memory impairment, "brain fog" Depressive syndrome, psychosis Stupor, coma Cerebellar ataxia, inner ear hearing loss Slowed reflexes
Musculoskeletal system
Muscle weakness, muscle hypotrophy, muscle pain, Elevation of the muscle enzyme creatine kinase Retarded bone growth in children
Gastrointestinal tract
Diminished appetite
Constipation
Megacolon, ileus (rare)
Ascites (rare)
Reproductive system
In women: menstrual irregularities, amenorrhoea, menorrhagia, infertility In men: reduced libido, impotence, gynaecomastia

(continued)

Table 7.1 (continued)

Metabolism
Reduced basal metabolic rate Weight gain Obesity High cholesterol, increased low-density lipoprotein (LDL), very low-density lipoprotein (VLDL), intermediate-density lipoprotein (IDL) and change in high-density lipoprotein (HDL) subclass Low glucose level
Other laboratory findings
Hyponatremia Anaemia Elevated creatine kinase

Onset and development of any complaints and symptoms
Permanent or temporary nature of symptoms
Change in neck size
Feeling a lump in one's throat, swallowing problems, feeling of tightness
Neck pain, hoarseness, voice change, distress
Fatigue, weight gain, cold intolerance
Hair and nail alterations
Changed eating habits and bowel movements
Eyelid oedema
Drug use
Use or discontinuation of any thyroid hormones, anti-thyroid drugs, amiodarone, interferon or other drugs potentially interfering with thyroid function
Iodine status
Recent application of contrast agents
Smoking
Comorbidity, history of other previous or current diseases

7.3 Physical Examination

Physical exam findings in hypothyroidism include:

A general impression suspicious of a hypothyroid state
Lack of motor functions, energy and agility
Pallor, tumidness
Inspection and palpation of the neck

- Scarring post-surgery
- Presence of a goitre or thyroid nodule
- Enlarged lymphatic nodes
- Neck size, neck pain, tenderness on palpation, pressor pain
- Stridor, congestion of neck veins

Hoarse voice and enlarged tongue
Retarded tendon reflexes
Dry and cold skin
Slower than normal heart rate and elevated blood pressure
Missing axillary hair as a sign of cortisol deficiency and secondary hypothyroidism
General examination and awareness of other diseases

7.4 Laboratory Thyroid Function Tests

Measurement of FT4 is regarded as the most sensitive test to diagnose overt hypothyroidism [3–5]. A confirmed low FT4 concentration is usually associated with a requirement of medical intervention and the oral substitution of thyroid hormones [6]. The free thyroid hormone FT4 can be reduced while the less accurate total T4 concentration may still be within its reference range [7]. If FT4 is low, the pituitary hormone TSH is expected to be markedly elevated in the diagnosis of primary hypothyroidism. This is however not true for *secondary or tertiary hypothyroidism*, where the TSH level may rather be low, normal or even slightly elevated, but in any event inappropriately low relative to the reduced FT4 concentration [8]. High levels of both TSH and FT4 hormones suggest, among other possibilities, the presence of resistance to thyroid hormone [9] (Table 7.2).

Table 7.2 Differential diagnosis of an elevated TSH value

Thyroid
Subclinical hypothyroidism Hypothyroidism
Pituitary
TSH-producing pituitary tumour
Adrenals
Adrenal insufficiency
Reduced sensitivity to thyroid hormone
Euthyroid thyroid hormone resistance syndromes Hypothyroid thyroid hormone resistance syndromes Selective resistance to T4 with normal T3 sensitivity TSH-receptor resistance
Low-T3 syndrome
Recovery phase
Methodological problems
Hysteresis, determination in non-equilibrium Assay interference HAMA (human anti-mouse antibody) interference Analytical error Pre-analytical error (blood clotting, poor storage of the sample) Sampling error

The combination of a high TSH concentration with an FT4 value still within its reference limits is classified by definition as *subclinical hypothyroidism* [6]. As discussed earlier, the *laboratory constellation*, however, does not allow the reliable diagnosis of a truly hypothyroid state of the patient, being *ambiguous* in its ethology, diagnostic implication and surrounded by uncertainty regarding its requirement of treatment. It may be useful as a screening test to indicate the presence of autoimmune thyroiditis, even though early thyroid failure may still be compensated, not requiring medical intervention at this stage. Long-term prognosis varies from return to normal, no change, to progression to overt hypothyroidism.

Thyroid hormones may be raised in the absence of TSH suppression. This constellation is equally *inappropriate*. It may be caused by levothyroxine treatment, TSH-secreting pituitary tumours, resistance to thyroid hormone β or α, MCT-8 deficiency, selenoprotein deficiency, analytical interference or measurements taken early in a non-equilibrated state [10].

FT3 is the *more active* sister hormone of FT4. As a result of its greater homeostatic stability in the physiological hypothalamic–pituitary–thyroid regulation, it is not closely correlated with either FT4 or TSH concentrations (see Chaps. 2 and 5). Accordingly, it warrants determination *in its own right*, in addition to the measurement of TSH and FT4. Assessment of FT3 and FT4 provides complementary and differentiated information. While FT4 is the main marker of hormone supply and thyroid failure in primary hypothyroidism, FT3 is a better indicator of thyroid hormone utilisation, and the ratio of the two hormones a measure of *balance between hormone supply and demand*. FT3 determination is especially useful in diagnosing forms of isolated *T3 hyperthyroidism* or *T3 thyrotoxicosis* due to levothyroxine overdosing and *inadequate substitution* with levothyroxine monotherapy due to *conversion inefficiency* in the utilisation of the precursor FT4. In addition, the evaluation of the FT3 to FT4 ratio or similar markers (SPINA-GD) has independent *prognostic value*, particularly for cardiovascular disease [11, 12].

In conditions, such as the low-T3 syndrome, where FT4 is not appropriately deiodinated at its outer ring to convert it to FT3 but preferentially deiodinated at the inner ring of the molecule, *reverse T3* (*rT3*) accumulates. Measurement of rT3 may be useful in special situations, although it is not routinely recommended in the diagnosis and treatment of hypothyroidism [13].

Methods and challenges of thyroid hormone measurements are discussed in a dedicated Chapter (see Chap. 8). An unresolved clinically challenging issue is a *lack of standardisation* among different assays commercially available for clinical use [14, 15]. This requires the individual laboratories to retest the applicability of manufacturer's recommendations and establish their own terms of reference for the thyroid function tests they provide [16–18]. This issue makes thyroid function tests not readily comparable across different platforms. Examples of typical reference ranges for the hormones are provided in Table 7.3. Those should not be regarded as universal, rather specific ranges provided by each laboratory must be considered. We also note that special situations require the use of more *specific reference ranges*, for instance reference intervals by trimester in pregnancy [19–25].

Table 7.3 Typical reference ranges for thyroid hormones

Thyroid-stimulating hormone (TSH)		
0.3–4 mIU/l		
Free thyroxine (FT4)		
10–25 pmol/l	0.8–2.0 ng/dl	Conversion factor 12.87
Free triiodothyronine (FT3)		
3.1–6.8 pmol/l	1.9–4.4 ng/dl	Conversion factor 1.54

The clinical interpretation of thyroid hormones depends heavily on patient *individuality and context* and is deeply embedded in the understanding of the hypothalamic–pituitary–thyroid axis regulation (Chap. 5). It goes far beyond the ordinary evaluation of other routine laboratory parameters. This can therefore only be appropriately done with the knowledge of the history and clinical condition of the patient and consideration of the *interrelated* nature of all thyroid parameters.

7.5 Ultrasonography of the Thyroid

Ultrasonography should be routinely included in the examination of a patient with a known or suspected thyroid disease. It directly allows the visualisation of the thyroid gland [26]. This may raise initial suspicion of the presence of *thyroid autoimmune disease*, for instance in a patient presenting with an ultrasonographic characteristic diffuse hypoechogenic pattern of the gland (Fig. 7.1).

A small or shrinking thyroid size may be another indicator of the disease.

The *volume* (ml) of the thyroid gland is determined by ultrasound according to the ellipsoid formula, with

Length × width × depth × 0.479 cm of each lobe
Addition of the lobe volumes, while the isthmus is not considered
Reference volume for adults, women < 18 and men < 25 ml
Reference values for children depend on age

The formula was derived from matching sonographic measurements with post-mortem investigations [27].

The assessment of the thyroid pattern and echogeneity is described as

Homogenous—inhomogenous,
Normal—hypoechogenic—hyperechogenic

Focal lesions, if present, should be detected, such as

local signs of inflammation—nodules—pseudonodules—lymphatic nodules
Cervical lymphatic nodes >1 cm are considered enlarged

The vascularisation of the thyroid gland using the Doppler mode warrants special attention, as

Increased vascularisation raises suspicion of Graves' disease
Reduced vascularisation raises suspicion of autoimmune thyroiditis

7.5.1 Shear Wave Elastography

Originally developed for the risk stratification of thyroid nodules, the technique of *shear wave elastography* proved valuable in the differential diagnosis of hypothyroidism. The method provides a quantitative method for the *stiffness* of the tissue, referred to as Young's module and measured in a unit of pressure (kPa) [28–30]. A value above 13 kPa supports the diagnosis of autoimmune thyroiditis (Fig. 6.1). In subacute thyroiditis, including COVID-19 thyroiditis, the results are usually higher than 100 kPa, whereas they use to be below 10 kPa in idiopathic hypothyroidism (e.g. due to TSH receptor mutations) [31].

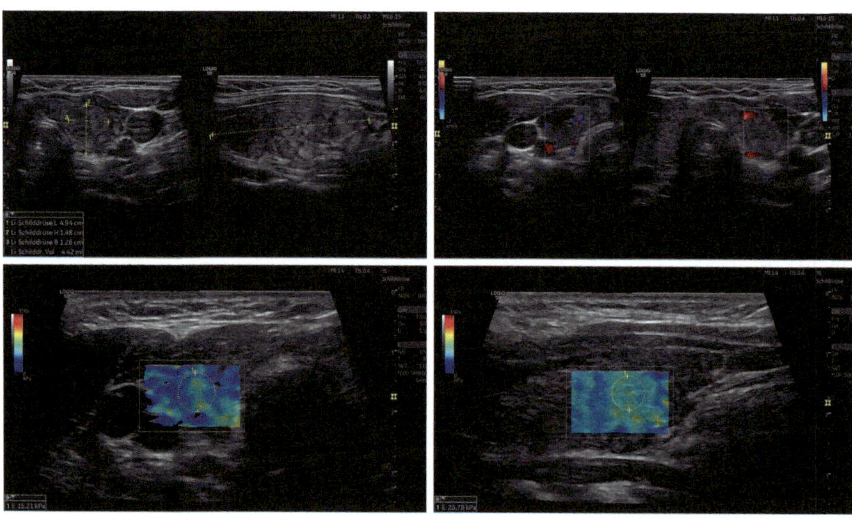

Fig. 7.1 Thyroid ultrasonographic image typical of autoimmune thyroiditis
This thyroid gland of a patient with autoimmune thyroiditis shows an inhomogeneous structure and typically hypoechogenic pattern (upper left panel) with low vascularisation in Duplex mode (upper right panel). Shear wave elastography adds further support for the presence of autoimmune thyroiditis (Young's module > 13 kPa) (lower panels)

7.6 Thyroid Scintigraphy

Technetium *scintigraphy* of the thyroid is not routinely required in the diagnostic work up of a patient with hypothyroidism [32]. Unlike morphological imaging by ultrasonography, scintigraphy produces an image of the functional activities across different areas of the thyroid gland including thyroid nodules.

The quantitative *technetium update* may be useful to differentiate between thyroiditis and Graves' disease, as it is low in the former and high in the latter.

The *distribution of the activity* in the thyroid differentiates between the presence of hyperfunctioning (hot, toxic adenoma) or hypofunctioning (cold) nodules. Cold nodules tend to show a higher rate of malignancies, compared to hot nodules. The combination of a toxic adenoma with autoimmune thyroid disease is known as Marine-Lenhart syndrome.

7.7 Fine Needle Aspiration

While not required in the diagnosis and treatment of hypothyroidism, in patients with additional thyroid nodules, which may raise a suspicion of malignancy, *fine needle aspiration* of the nodule should be performed [33]. Related to autoimmune thyroiditis and hypothyroidism is the occasional presence of lymphomas, which should also undergo fine needle aspiration for diagnostic purpose.

7.8 Cardiac Tests

Cardiac manifestations of hypothyroidism are frequent [34]. Electrocardiogram (ECG) is therefore a routine procedure to document possible abnormalities in heart beat and cardiac arrhythmia in thyroid patients. While atrial fibrillation occurs frequently in association with hyperthyroidism, typical signs of hypothyroidism in ECG include bradycardia and a prolonged QT interval. In severe cases higher-grade abnormalities of the cardiac conduction system have been observed [35]. ECG may also be required to monitor hypothyroid patients on levothyroxine treatment, particularly in patients susceptible to atrial fibrillation. *Echocardiography* aids in more specific conditions occasionally found in hypothyroid patients including pericardial effusion or an impaired ejection fraction.

7.9 Quality of Life Assessment

Patient-reported outcomes are increasingly integrated into clinical practice [36]. They may improve the quality of care, structure the physician–patient communication and enhance patient satisfaction [37]. Their use in the care for thyroid patients has been facilitated by the availability of validated thyroid-specific quality-of-life scales, such as the *ThyPRO questionnaire* [38–42]. They have been reported to improve symptomatic management and communication with patients. These instruments are also used to compare quality of care across disease entities, treatment modalities, institutions and geographical regions [39, 42, 43]. The lengthy questionnaires are preferably answered electronically by patients due to their time-consuming nature and risk of inadvertent errors. The retrospective surveys have a limited time window with a recall period of 1–4 weeks [44]. It is well known that patients with benign thyroid diseases report short- and long-term impairments in their *quality of life* [45]. What is less clear is their causal relationship with thyroid function and the underlying thyroid disease, as opposed to non-specific influences, such as pre-existing or subsequent comorbidity and patient expectations. Notably, the impairment in the quality of life does not appear to be positively correlated with the severity of hypothyroidism, even an inverse association has been reported in a small sample [46]. However, patients who showed a decrease in FT3 index following treatment scored significantly worse in this study [46]. Hence, the thresholds may not be the same in health and disease. Although some issues are currently not resolved, the instruments help identify areas of concern to be discussed and addressed.

References

1. Hörmann R. Schilddrüsenkrankheiten: Leitfaden für Praxis und Klinik. Berlin: ABW Wissenschaftsverlag; 2005. p. 1–268.
2. Bogdan C, Ivan VM, Apostol A, Sandu OE, Maralescu FM, Lighezan DF. Hypothyroidism and heart rate variability: implications for cardiac autonomic regulation. Diagnostics (Basel). 2024;14:1261. https://doi.org/10.3390/diagnostics14121261.
3. Baloch Z, Carayon P, Conte-Devolx B, Demers LM, Feldt-Rasmussen U, Henry JF, Livosli VA, Niccoli-Sire P, John R, Ruf J, Smyth PP, Spencer CA, Stockigt JR, Guidelines Committee NAOCB. Laboratory medicine practice guidelines. Laboratory support for the diagnosis and monitoring of thyroid disease. Thyroid. 2004;13:3–126. https://doi.org/10.1089/105072503321086962.
4. Spencer CA. Laboratory thyroid tests: a historical perspective. Thyroid. 2023;33:407–19. https://doi.org/10.1089/thy.2022.0397.
5. Van Uytfanghe K, Ehrenkranz J, Halsall D, Hoff K, Loh TP, Spencer CA, Köhrle J. Thyroid stimulating hormone and thyroid hormones (triiodothyronine and thyroxine): an American Thyroid Association-commissioned review of current clinical and laboratory status. Thyroid. 2023;33:1013–28. https://doi.org/10.1089/thy.2023.0169.
6. Jonklaas J, Bianco AC, Bauer AJ, Burman KD, Cappola AR, Celi FS, Cooper DS, Kim BW, Peeters RP, Rosenthal MS, Sawka AM. Guidelines for the treatment of hypothyroidism: prepared by the American Thyroid Association task force on thyroid hormone replacement. Thyroid. 2014;24:1670–751. https://doi.org/10.1089/thy.2014.0028.
7. Midgley JEM. Direct and indirect free thyroxine assay methods: theory and practice. Clin Chem. 2001;47:1353–63.
8. Beck-Peccoz P, Rodari G, Giavoli C, Lania A. Central hypothyroidism—a neglected thyroid disorder. Nat Rev Endocrinol. 2017;13:588–98. https://doi.org/10.1038/nrendo.2017.47.

9. Grasberger H, Refetoff S. Resistance to thyrotropin. Best Pract Res Clin Endocrinol Metab. 2017;31:183–94. https://doi.org/10.1016/j.beem.2017.03.004.
10. Moran C, Schoenmakers N, Halsall D, Oddy S, Lyons G, Van Den Berg S, Gurnell M, Chatterjee K. Approach to the patient with raised thyroid hormones and nonsuppressed TSH. J Clin Endocrinol Metab. 2024;109:1094–108. https://doi.org/10.1210/clinem/dgad681.
11. Lang X, Li Y, Zhang D, Zhang Y, Wu N, Zhang Y. FT3 to FT4 ratio is correlated with all-cause mortality, cardiovascular mortality, and cardiovascular disease risk: NHANES 2007-2012. Front Endocrinol (Lausanne). 2022;13:964822. https://doi.org/10.3389/fendo.2022.964822.
12. Müller P, Leow MK, Dietrich JW. Minor perturbations of thyroid homeostasis and major cardiovascular endpoints-physiological mechanisms and clinical evidence. Front Cardiovasc Med. 2022;9:942971. https://doi.org/10.3389/fcvm.2022.942971.
13. Schmidt RL, Lopresti JS, Mcdermott MT, Zick SM, Straseski JA. Does reverse triiodothyronine testing have clinical utility? An analysis of practice variation based on order data from a national reference laboratory. Thyroid. 2018;28:842–8. https://doi.org/10.1089/thy.2017.0645.
14. Thienpont LM, Van Uytfanghe K, Beastall G, Faix JD, Ieiri T, Miller WG, Nelson JC, Ronin C, Ross HA, Thijssen JH, Toussaint B, Tests IFCCWGOSOTF. Report of the IFCC working group for standardization of thyroid function tests; part 2: free thyroxine and free triiodothyronine. Clin Chem. 2010;56:912–20. https://doi.org/10.1373/clinchem.2009.140194.
15. Thienpont LM, Van Uytfanghe K, Beastall G, Faix JD, Ieiri T, Miller WG, Nelson JC, Ronin C, Ross HA, Thijssen JH, Toussaint B, Tests IFCCWGOSOTF. Report of the IFCC working group for standardization of thyroid function tests; part 1: thyroid-stimulating hormone. Clin Chem. 2010;56:902–11. https://doi.org/10.1373/clinchem.2009.140178.
16. Wayne PA. Clinical and laboratory standards institute: performance standards for antimicrobial susceptibility testing: 20th informational supplement. CLSI Document. 2010:M100–S20.
17. Larisch R, Giacobino A, Eckl WA, Wahl HG, Midgley JEM, Hoermann R. Reference range for thyrotropin. Post hoc assessment. Nuklearmedizin. 2015;54:112–7. https://doi.org/10.3413/Nukmed-0671-14-06.
18. De Grande LAC, Van Uytfanghe K, Reynders D, Das B, Faix JD, Mackenzie F, Decallonne B, Hishinuma A, Lapauw B, Taelman P, Van Crombrugge P, Van Den Bruel A, Velkeniers B, Williams P, Thienpont LM. Standardization of free thyroxine measurements allows the adoption of a more uniform reference interval. Clin Chem. 2017;63:1642–52. https://doi.org/10.1373/clinchem.2017.274407.
19. Stricker R, Echenard M, Eberhart R, Chevailler M-C, Perez V, Quinn FA, Stricker R. Evaluation of maternal thyroid function during pregnancy: the importance of using gestational age-specific reference intervals. Eur J Endocrinol. 2007;157:509–14. https://doi.org/10.1530/EJE-07-0249.
20. Laurberg P, Andersen SL, Hindersson P, Nohr EA, Olsen J. Dynamics and predictors of serum TSH and FT4 reference limits in early pregnancy: a study within the Danish national birth cohort. J Clin Endocrinol Metab. 2016;101:2484–92. https://doi.org/10.1210/jc.2016-1387.
21. Derakhshan A, Shu H, Broeren MAC, De Poortere RA, Wikström S, Peeters RP, Demeneix B, Bornehag CG, Korevaar TIM. Reference ranges and determinants of thyroid function during early pregnancy: the Selma study. J Clin Endocrinol Metab. 2018;103:3548–56. https://doi.org/10.1210/jc.2018-00890.
22. Gao X, Li Y, Li J, Liu A, Sun W, Teng W, Shan Z. Gestational TSH and FT4 reference intervals in Chinese women: a systematic review and meta-analysis. Front Endocrinol (Lausanne). 2018;9:432. https://doi.org/10.3389/fendo.2018.00432.
23. Andersen SL, Christensen PA, Knøsgaard L, Andersen S, Handberg A, Hansen AB, Vestergaard P. Classification of thyroid dysfunction in pregnant women differs by analytical method and type of thyroid function test. J Clin Endocrinol Metab. 2020;105:dgaa567. https://doi.org/10.1210/clinem/dgaa567.
24. Pop VJ, Hulsbosch LP, Boekhorst MGBM, Broeren MAC, Krabbe JG, Wiersinga WM. Hypothyroid symptoms throughout pregnancy are predominantly associated with thyroxine and not with thyrotropin concentrations. Thyroid. 2022;32:1249–58. https://doi.org/10.1089/thy.2022.0244.

25. Osinga JAJ, Derakhshan A, Feldt-Rasmussen U, Huang K, Vrijkotte TGM, Männistö T, Bassols J, López-Bermejo A, Aminorroaya A, Vafeiadi M, Broeren MAC, Palomaki GE, Ashoor G, Chen L, Lu X, Taylor PN, Tao FB, Brown SJ, Sitoris G, Chatzi L, Vaidya B, Popova PV, Vasukova EA, Kianpour M, Suvanto E, Grineva EN, Hattersley A, Pop VJM, Nelson SM, Walsh JP, Nicolaides KH, D'alton ME, Poppe KG, Chaker L, Bliddal S, Korevaar TIM. TSH and FT4 reference interval recommendations and prevalence of gestational thyroid dysfunction: quantification of current diagnostic approaches. J Clin Endocrinol Metab. 2024;109:868–78. https://doi.org/10.1210/clinem/dgad564.
26. Quadbeck B, Wawrzyn H, Saller B, Hormann R, Mann K. Sonography of the thyroid gland. Med Welt. 2001;52:28–32.
27. Brunn J, Block U, Ruf G, Bos I, Kunze WP, Scriba PC. Volumetric analysis of thyroid lobes by real-time ultrasound (author's transl). Dtsch Med Wochenschr. 1981;106:1338–40. https://doi.org/10.1055/s-2008-1070506.
28. Hazem M, Al Jabr IK, Alyahya AA, Hassanein AG, Algahlan HAE. Reliability of shear wave elastography in the evaluation of diffuse thyroid diseases in children and adolescents. Eur J Radiol. 2021;143:109942. https://doi.org/10.1016/j.ejrad.2021.109942.
29. Kara T, Ateş F, Durmaz MS, Akyürek N, Durmaz FG, Özbakır B, Öztürk M. Assessment of thyroid gland elasticity with shear-wave elastography in Hashimoto's thyroiditis patients. J Ultrasound. 2020;23:543–51. https://doi.org/10.1007/s40477-020-00437-y.
30. Decker T, Schnittka E, Stolzenberg L, Yalowitz J. Shear-wave elastography for the diagnosis of pediatric Hashimoto's thyroiditis: a systematic review and meta-analysis. Cureus. 2023;15:e35490. https://doi.org/10.7759/cureus.35490.
31. Golu I, Balas M, Amzar D, Milos I, Corlan A, Vlad M. The value of shear-wave elastography in the diagnosis and follow-up of post covid-19 subacute thyroiditis. Ultrasound Med Biol. 2022;48:S44. (Abstract)
32. Giovanella L, Avram AM, Iakovou I, Kwak J, Lawson SA, Lulaj E, Luster M, Piccardo A, Schmidt M, Tulchinsky M, Verburg FA, Wolin E. EANM practice guideline/SNMMI procedure standard for RAIU and thyroid scintigraphy. Eur J Nucl Med Mol Imaging. 2019;46:2514–25. https://doi.org/10.1007/s00259-019-04472-8.
33. Paschke R, Cantara S, Crescenzi A, Jarzab B, Musholt TJ, Sobrinho Simoes M. European Thyroid Association guidelines regarding thyroid nodule molecular fine-needle aspiration cytology diagnostics. Eur Thyroid J. 2017;6:115–29. https://doi.org/10.1159/000468519.
34. Kahaly GJ, Dillmann WH. Thyroid hormone action in the heart. Endocr Rev. 2005;26:704–28.
35. Chatzitomaris A, Scheeler M, Gotzmann M, Köditz R, Schildroth J, Knyhala KM, Nicolas V, Heyer C, Mügge A, Klein HH, Dietrich JW. Second degree av block and severely impaired contractility in cardiac myxedema: a case report. Thyroid Res. 2015;8:6. https://doi.org/10.1186/s13044-015-0018-2.
36. Cramon PK, Bjorner JB, Groenvold M, Boesen VB, Bonnema SJ, Hegedüs L, Feldt-Rasmussen U, Rasmussen ÅK, Watt T. Implementation of thyroid-related patient-reported outcomes in routine clinical practice. Front Endocrinol (Lausanne). 2022;13:1000682. https://doi.org/10.3389/fendo.2022.1000682.
37. Chan EKH, Edwards TC, Haywood K, Mikles SP, Newton L. Implementing patient-reported outcome measures in clinical practice: a companion guide to the isoqol user's guide. Qual Life Res. 2019;28:621–7. https://doi.org/10.1007/s11136-018-2048-4.
38. Watt T, Hegedüs L, Groenvold M, Bjorner JB, Rasmussen AK, Bonnema SJ, Feldt-Rasmussen U. Validity and reliability of the novel thyroid-specific quality of life questionnaire, thypro. Eur J Endocrinol. 2010;162:161–7. https://doi.org/10.1530/EJE-09-0521.
39. Watt T, Cramon P, Hegedüs L, Bjorner JB, Bonnema SJ, Rasmussen ÅK, Feldt-Rasmussen U, Groenvold M. The thyroid-related quality of life measure thypro has good responsiveness and ability to detect relevant treatment effects. J Clin Endocrinol Metab. 2014;99:3708–17. https://doi.org/10.1210/jc.2014-1322.

40. Watt T, Bjorner JB, Groenvold M, Cramon P, Winther KH, Hegedüs L, Bonnema SJ, Rasmussen ÅK, Ware JE, Feldt-Rasmussen U. Development of a short version of the thyroid-related patient-reported outcome thypro. Thyroid. 2015;25:1069–79. https://doi.org/10.1089/thy.2015.0209.
41. Winther KH, Cramon P, Watt T, Bjorner JB, Ekholm O, Feldt-Rasmussen U, Groenvold M, Rasmussen ÅK, Hegedüs L, Bonnema SJ. Disease-specific as well as generic quality of life is widely impacted in autoimmune hypothyroidism and improves during the first six months of levothyroxine therapy. PLoS One. 2016;11:e0156925. https://doi.org/10.1371/journal.pone.0156925.
42. Larisch R, Midgley JEM, Dietrich JW, Hoermann R. Effect of radioiodine treatment on quality of life in patients with subclinical hyperthyroidism: a prospective controlled study. In: NuclaearMedicine, Larisch R, Midgley JEM, Dietrich JW, Hoermann R, editors. Effect of radioiodine treatment on quality of life in patients with subclinical hyperthyroidism: a prospective controlled study, vol. 63. NuclearMedicine; 2024. p. 176–87. https://doi.org/10.1055/a-2240-8087.
43. Törring O, Watt T, Sjölin G, Byström K, Abraham-Nordling M, Calissendorff J, Cramon PK, Filipsson Nyström H, Hallengren B, Holmberg M, Khamisi S, Lantz M, Wallin G. Impaired quality of life after radioiodine therapy compared to antithyroid drugs or surgical treatment for Graves' hyperthyroidism: a long-term follow-up with the thyroid-related patient-reported outcome questionnaire and 36-item short form health status survey. Thyroid. 2019;29:322–31. https://doi.org/10.1089/thy.2018.0315.
44. Boesen VB, Feldt-Rasmussen U, Bjorner JB, Cramon PK, Grøenvold M, Rasmussen ÅK, Watt T. Shorter recall period for the thyroid-related patient-reported outcome measure Thypro did not change the accuracy as evaluated by repeated momentary measurements. Thyroid. 2020;30:185–91. https://doi.org/10.1089/thy.2019.0380.
45. Watt T, Groenvold M, Rasmussen ÅK, Bonnema SJ, Hegedüs L, Bjorner JB, Feldt-Rasmussen U. Quality of life in patients with benign thyroid disorders. A review. Eur J Endocrinol. 2006;154:501–10. https://doi.org/10.1530/eje.1.02124.
46. Larsen CB, Winther KH, Cramon PK, Rasmussen ÅK, Feldt-Rasmussen U, Groenvold M, Bjorner JB, Hegedüs L, Watt T, Bonnema SJ. Severity of hypothyroidism is inversely associated with impaired quality of life in patients referred to an endocrine clinic. Thyroid Res. 2023;16:37. https://doi.org/10.1186/s13044-023-00178-0.

Chapter 8
Biochemical Thyroid Function Testing

Rudolf Hoermann and Johannes W. Dietrich

Biochemical testing is a cornerstone in the management of hypothyroidism. Laboratory thyroid tests have seen impressive technical advances over the past decades [1–3]. They are essential for the accurate diagnosis of thyroid disorders because signs and symptoms of the disease are frequently subtle in many patients with hypothyroidism, making biochemical testing necessary to detect and/or confirm the disease [4]. This view has been taken one step further, leading to the introduction of an entirely new category of disease, *subclinical hypothyroidism*, and its counterpart subclinical hyperthyroidism [5]. The definition of disease has thereby been *separated* from the clinical expression of any signs and symptoms of a thyroid dysfunction and is solely based on biochemical testing. It relies on the reliability of the measurement of TSH as the presumed single most sensitive thyroid parameter. In Chap. 5 we thoroughly examined and questioned this practice on the basis of an improved and extended understanding of hypothalamic–pituitary–thyroid regulation. This *redefines* the role of TSH in the thyroid system and, consequently, as a

R. Hoermann (✉)
Yandina, QLD, Australia

Department of General Internal Medicine, Gastroenterology and Endocrinology, [Retired] Klinikum Lüdenscheid, Lüdenscheid, Germany
e-mail: rudolf.hoermann@gmail.com

J. W. Dietrich
Diabetes, Endocrinology and Metabolism Section, Department of Medicine, St. Josef-Hospital, Ruhr University Hospitals, Bochum, Germany

Centre for Diabetes Technology (ZDT), Catholic Hospitals Bochum, Bochum, Germany

Centre for Rare Endocrine Diseases (ZSEK), Ruhr Center for Rare Diseases (CeSER), Ruhr University of Bochum and Witten/Herdecke University, Bochum, Germany

Centre for Thyroid Medicine (ZSM), Ruhr University of Bochum, Bochum, Germany
e-mail: johannes.dietrich@ruhr-uni-bochum.de

R. Hoermann, J. W. Dietrich (eds.), *Hypothyroidism*,
https://doi.org/10.1007/978-981-96-3682-2_8

clinical utility. The focus has recently shifted back from an over-reliance on TSH to the need of direct measurement of thyroid hormones [6–9]. In Chap. 9, we take a closer look at the quality of the methods used for thyroid function testing, choice of hormones to be tested and assays best suited for optimisation of the diagnostic process.

References

1. Baloch Z, Carayon P, Conte-Devolx B, Demers LM, Feldt-Rasmussen U, Henry JF, Livosli VA, Niccoli-Sire P, John R, Ruf J, Smyth PP, Spencer CA, Stockigt JR, Guidelines Committee NAOCB. Laboratory medicine practice guidelines. Laboratory support for the diagnosis and monitoring of thyroid disease. Thyroid. 2004;13:3–126. https://doi.org/10.1089/105072503321086962.
2. Spencer CA. Laboratory thyroid tests: a historical perspective. Thyroid. 2023;33:407–19. https://doi.org/10.1089/thy.2022.0397.
3. Van Uytfanghe K, Ehrenkranz J, Halsall D, Hoff K, Loh TP, Spencer CA, Köhrle J. Thyroid stimulating hormone and thyroid hormones (triiodothyronine and thyroxine): an American Thyroid Association-commissioned review of current clinical and laboratory status. Thyroid. 2023;33:1013–28. https://doi.org/10.1089/thy.2023.0169.
4. Jansen HI, Boelen A, Heijboer AC, Bruinstroop E, Fliers E. Hypothyroidism: the difficulty in attributing symptoms to their underlying cause. Front Endocrinol (Lausanne). 2023;14:1130661. https://doi.org/10.3389/fendo.2023.1130661.
5. Jonklaas J, Bianco AC, Bauer AJ, Burman KD, Cappola AR, Celi FS, Cooper DS, Kim BW, Peeters RP, Rosenthal MS, Sawka AM. Guidelines for the treatment of hypothyroidism: prepared by the American Thyroid Association task force on thyroid hormone replacement. Thyroid. 2014;24:1670–751. https://doi.org/10.1089/thy.2014.0028.
6. Hoermann R, Midgley JEM, Larisch R, Dietrich JW. Individualised requirements for optimum treatment of hypothyroidism: complex needs, limited options. Drugs Context. 2019;8:212597. https://doi.org/10.7573/dic.212597.
7. Fitzgerald SP, Bean NG, Hennessey JV, Falhammar H. Thyroid testing paradigm switch from thyrotropin to thyroid hormones-future directions and opportunities in clinical medicine and research. Endocrine. 2021;74:285–9. https://doi.org/10.1007/s12020-021-02851-6.
8. Fitzgerald SP, Falhammar H. Redefinition of successful treatment of patients with hypothyroidism. Is TSH the best biomarker of euthyroidism. Front Endocrinol (Lausanne). 2022;13:920854. https://doi.org/10.3389/fendo.2022.920854.
9. Lawton RI, Sabatini BL, Hochbaum DR. Longevity, demographic characteristics, and socio-economic status are linked to triiodothyronine levels in the general population. Proc Natl Acad Sci USA. 2024;121(2):e2308652121. https://doi.org/10.1073/pnas.2308652121.

Chapter 9
The New Paradigm for Thyroid Function Diagnosis and Treatment: Conceptual and Technical Barriers to Consistent Outcomes

John E. Midgley, Rudolf Hoermann, and Johannes W. Dietrich

9.1 Introduction

Recent discoveries have challenged the diagnostic dominance of thyroid-stimulating hormone (TSH), especially in treatment of hypothyroid patients with oral thyroid hormone. The prominent role of free thyroid hormone assay (FT4 and FT3) measurements as determinants of satisfactory treatment in themselves or through a ratio as an indicator of T4 conversion to T3 is now beginning to be recognised after a long period of relative neglect. The new findings inform the best way to regain health,

---

The author "John E Midgley" died after approving his chapter prior to the submission of the book. This is one of his last works.

J. E. Midgley (✉)
North Lakes Clinical, Ilkley, UK

R. Hoermann
Yandina, QLD, Australia

Department of General Internal Medicine, Gastroenterology and Endocrinology, [Retired] Klinikum Lüdenscheid, Lüdenscheid, Germany
e-mail: rudolf.hoermann@gmail.com

J. W. Dietrich
Diabetes, Endocrinology and Metabolism Section, Department of Medicine, St. Josef-Hospital, Ruhr University Hospitals, Bochum, Germany

Centre for Diabetes Technology (ZDT), Catholic Hospitals Bochum, Bochum, Germany

Centre for Rare Endocrine Diseases (ZSEK), Ruhr Center for Rare Diseases (CeSER), Ruhr University of Bochum and Witten/Herdecke University, Bochum, Germany

Centre for Thyroid Medicine (ZSM), Ruhr University of Bochum, Bochum, Germany
e-mail: johannes.dietrich@ruhr-uni-bochum.de

R. Hoermann, J. W. Dietrich (eds.), *Hypothyroidism*,
https://doi.org/10.1007/978-981-96-3682-2_9

when combined with the equally key role of patient presentation. In order to rehearse the developments that have led to this re-evaluation, this chapter is devoted to a narrative on the history of thyroid function diagnosis and the tests used to optimise medication for hypothyroidism. It is to be read in the light of arguments elsewhere in this book that re-examine the physiology of thyroid function and malfunction and its effect on the choice of diagnosis and treatment. I shall initially comment briefly on progress in these activities from the viewpoint of a physical chemist/biochemist and inventor of the labelled one-step analogue and labelled antibody-free thyroid hormone assays currently used routinely. Since 1985, the sensitive TSH assay has become a powerful (and sometimes claimed as only needed) determinant of hypothyroidism and satisfactory treatment. However, the hitherto dominant role of sensitive TSH assays in controlling therapy has become suspect. Accordingly, in therapy for hormone supplementation, it is becoming clear that the role of TSH has been overstated and the free thyroid hormone assays (FT4 and FT3) play far more important and decisive roles in the diagnostic process. Consequently, the consistency of their performance has become a key determinant of their diagnostic value. Regrettably, it appears that, while TSH assays have been better, though not completely, harmonised, FT4 and especially FT3 assays from different manufacturers still display considerable variability in performance. Almost all do not obey the fundamental requirements that demonstrate satisfactory performance. There is little doubt that, unlike the perceived need for accurate TSH testing, failure to similarly redesign FT4/FT3 test performance has led to a loss of impetus owing to the overwhelming dominance of TSH as a favoured diagnostic. Given the present situation, this highlights the shortcomings of regulators and manufacturers of such assays, which have permitted their inconsistent measurements. In addition, historical allegations of basic inadequacy of the underlying technique have arisen, consequently becoming unquestioned certainties embedded in the literature. These false criticisms have sharply illuminated the lack of physical chemistry understanding underlying these methods. The basic fallacies of these allegations are revealed here. In addition, the paucity of reported use of assays, which are soundly based, invites further comment on why they do not figure more frequently in the literature. The influence of integrated diagnostic platforms and the resulting restriction of an individual choice of tests are postulated as contributing factors. It would also seem that in addition financial considerations may dominate platform choice, together with the apparent indifference of users (other than complaint as to the quality of the products they engage with). Finally, I make suggestions as to how this presently unsatisfactory state of affairs could be improved.

9.2 Thyroid Hormone Testing: Where Have We Come From?

This section comprises a brief history of the development of thyroid treatment from its empirical beginnings to the present day. The dawn of modern treatment of thyroid dysfunction dates back to [1] when sheep thyroid extract was injected into sufferers having lost glandular function. This was later succeeded by oral uptake of pig thyroid extract [2]. Problems immediately arose in that (a) there were no suitable tests other than patient response to monitor recovery of health and (b) the products themselves were variable in hormone content. Significant advances were made in determining the molecular structures of T4, which was discovered in 1927, and T3 [3, 4]. This understanding of the nature of these two molecules could permit the later development of suitable specific assays. However, the then existing American Pharmacopeia was based on quality control on iodine content only, without further separation of different hormone species. This was reviewed in the 1985 edition and products with a more precisely measured T4 and T3 content were now required. A comprehensive discourse on the history of detection and treatment of dysfunction is available [5, 6].

The history of the development of blood tests for dysfunction began with the production of a protein-bound iodine (PBI) measurement [7, 8]. Though this dealt reasonably well with a large number of patients, it could not resolve the contributions of T4 and T3. It was also at fault in that the PBI value was affected by individual patient variation in the serum concentration of the T4-/T3-binding proteins. For example, the primary thyroxine-binding globulin (TBG) concentrations can vary from 0 (TBG deficiency) up to 5 times the mean reference range value [9]. Hence the measurement of the total hormone levels can fluctuate in a parallel fashion. Additionally, the test could not be used to measure the important free (unbound) fraction of T4 which was realised to be the principal determinant of health. Interference from iodine of a non-thyroidal origin was also a significant problem [8].

In addressing this problem, a radioactive assay based on the competitive binding of ambient and radio-labelled T4 to the serum-binding proteins was produced for total hormone measurement [10], together with a second test (T3 uptake) which was designed to correct for a patient's individual T4-binding protein concentrations [11]. Though going some way to resolving the difficulties, the basic misunderstanding of the T3 uptake test's mode of working caused some problems in the interpretation of results. This was especially prominent in the results in late pregnancy, where fortuitously the uptake test corrected them as having FT4 concentrations closely equivalent to a non-pregnant cohort [12]. This is now known to be an artefact [13, 14] but was for a long time strongly though invalidly regarded as being a better measurement [12]. Nevertheless, inadequate FT4 assays can erroneously show overestimated FT4 values in late pregnancy [15]. However, given that the uptake test has long been shown to be unsound [14], it is remarkable and rather dispiriting that this test is still used today.

With the discoveries of the molecular structure of T4 and T3 [3, 4] and the later development of immunoassays for total T4 and T3 (T4- and T3-IA), better accuracy and precision could be achieved [16, 17]. Somewhat earlier, an immunoassay for thyrotropin (TSH) was developed [18]. Its use of polyclonal antibody as a probe restricted it to diagnosing hypothyroidism, since it was not sensitive enough, because of the antibody's heterogeneous nature, to detect the low values typical of hyperthyroidism [19]. For a while, the combination of these assays with T3 uptake continued, but the shortcomings of the latter propelled a need for direct measurement of the free (unbound) fractions that determined thyroid status. In the late 1970's and early 1980s, two major developments became available to solve the problem. One was a two-step method [20] in which serum is first incubated with an immobilised T4 antibody. Then, after discarding the liquid, a marker T4 is introduced to give an estimate of FT4. The problem with this method is (a) it requires extra steps, which affects precision and (b) if the antibody probe binding is too weak, there is always the possibility of a back-reaction releasing T4 in the subsequent serum-free incubation with tracer.

An alternative method was developed at the same time. This used an analogue of T4 (T3) whose essential property is to bind strongly to the appropriate antibody, but much less if at all to the serum-binding proteins [21, 22]. This approach has the advantage that the procedure is basically identical to a total T4 assay in the steps required and the achievable precision. The earliest FT4 (FT3) assays were successful at eliminating effects from T4 bound to TBG and transthyretin, but a small influence of albumin remained [22, 23]. This prompted multiple attempts to discredit the technique [24–26], even though the effects were only significant in non-thyroidal illness and familial dysalbuminemic hyperthyroxinaemia (FDH) [27], the former of which was at that time termed "euthyroid sick syndrome" with the connotations for expected FT4 concentrations that implied [24]. Now this problem is known to be far more variable as regards function test values and gives different results unique to the situation [28]. The first false allegation of significant shortcomings of these assays emanated from the effects of adding albumin in vitro. This work apparently bolstered the perceived reality of the "albumin effect" [24–26]. However, it was shown to be invalid as a means to quantitate any effect on the FT4 assay, as the responses to added albumin varied widely according to its source and purity [29]. In the first tests there were also problems with hormone-bearing autoantibodies, but a secondary test was devised to detect such patients and diagnose accordingly [30]. Various allegations of significant general faults in the one-step direct FT4/3 assays were made over a long period (even questioning their basic validity). All these are ill-founded as will be discussed later. The essential need for an improvement of analogue one-step assays, at least to nullify serum albumin interference, led to a test module that, while remaining one-step, shifted the assay tracer probe onto the antibody itself [31, 32]. An immobilised poly-molecular competitor then competed with FT4/FT3 for binding with the antibody. It was also thought to be useful if interference from serum autoantibodies could be minimised [31, 32]. Hence, for an FT4 assay, instead of using a poly-molecular T4, a corresponding T3 derivative was used. This took advantage of the weak cross-reactivity of the T4 antibody with the T3 acceptor, in that a large excess was needed to produce a satisfactory FT4 dose curve. This excess could now accommodate serum T4 or T3 autoantibodies, without significantly affecting the antibody tracer's binding ability [34]. This combination successfully removed serum albumin dependency from the assay, and minimised autoantibody interference [32]. This method constituted the one-step Amerlex-MAB FT4 assay, which was first introduced with a radioactive tracer but culminated in a non-radioactive equivalent [33, 34]. A similar FT3 assay was also produced, but used a labelled T3 antibody with an immobilised T2 polymer as competitor for binding with FT3.

As mentioned earlier, initial assays for TSH were incapable of directly measuring the suppressed level of the hormone typical of hyperthyroidism. Thus, for a short while, patient presentation remained as a necessary adjunct to biochemical measurements. However, in 1985 monoclonal antibody-based TSH assays achieved accurate measurement over the whole spectrum of thyroid function and now, after further improvement, have become exquisitely sensitive [19]. Unfortunately, the looked-for harmonisation of results between various measuring platforms has still not been satisfactorily achieved [35]. Nevertheless, the high sensitivity of the TSH test encouraged its present position as the test of choice over FT4 [36]. Especially this was the case in treatment for hypothyroidism, where it is still believed that, in nearly all cases, oral T4 alone can fully restore the appropriate conversion to T3, and, by simple feedback control shown by a TSH value in its reference range, will satisfactorily demonstrate correct dosage [36]. This thinking has crystallised over the past 38 years—normalisation of the TSH value has become the primary decisive aim for adequate replacement. Usually, FT3 assays are often only used to detect hyperthyroidism.

9.3 Thyroid Function Testing: Where Are We Now?

As indicated above, the great sensitivity of TSH compared with other tests has led diagnosticians to promote its dominance over FT4 and FT3 [19, 36]. But great sensitivity is not inevitably correlated with great utility. Many FT4 and FT3 tests remain much as they were, in terms of the shortcomings that persist in many such assays. However, several comments can be made about the problems from the blind use of statistics and the resulting diagnoses which are in evidence today. For example, it is the norm to express the reference range of an analyte as enclosing 95% of values within its limits. Especially in the case of TSH, the reference range displays a strongly skewed distribution, requiring normalisation by logarithmic transformation [37]. The reasons why this right-hand skew exists have been frequently aired and the exact state of patients with TSH values high in the skew distribution have been questioned [37–40]. Routinely the 95% reference range used as a statistical cut-off omits about 2.5% of the so-called euthyroid patients below the low reference line, and 2.5% above the high limit. Owing to the long "tail" of subjects omitted in the upper reaches, one has to ask, in what category such persons are to be placed? Adding both ends of the scale, a total of 5% of subjects are cast into limbo, with the upper echelon being spread quite widely. Are these patients to be considered euthyroid or subclinically hypo(hyper)thyroid patients? This conundrum demonstrates the error of diagnosing patients merely by statistical placement. This has encouraged another statistically based decision to view values up to 10 units as indicating subclinical hypothyroidism and not therefore generally requiring treatment. This approach is claimed to minimise overlapping diagnostic complexity, thus also minimising the number of false-positives/negatives [41, 42]. But it is still the case that some individuals in this shadowy region may really be truly hypothyroid and in need of treatment. This shows an insoluble problem, raised by diagnosing by statistics instead of presentation. Indeed, the whole concept of subclinical hypothyroidism, by being cast as a statistical moiety in itself, is of doubtful validity. It may alternatively be due to a constellation of thyroidal and non-thyroidal effects.

It is now, however reluctantly, slowly dawning on the thyroid community that diagnosis and treatment control with TSH have lacked authenticity over the past 38 years when the sensitive test has overridden all before it. The control mechanisms of the hypothalamic–pituitary–thyroid (HPT) axis are far more complex than previously thought and deny the simple feedback models [43–45] that define universally satisfactory treatment by T4 alone. A minority of patients also may require T3 in addition, not simply to raise serum FT4 but also FT3 levels. The thyroidal feed-forward T3 shunt has made the assumed universally satisfactory T4-T3 conversion from T4 alone to be in error in the athyreotic subject. This subject is discussed in more detail in other chapters.

9.4 Fallacies in Opposing Free Thyroid Hormone Test Validity

Criticisms of the fidelity especially of one-step FT4 and FT3 assays have come from four directions. In the first such assays, there was without doubt a certain minor effect of serum albumin in the results, only evident in the low-albumin state of non-thyroidal illness. This was allegedly demonstrated in two ways. First, as discussed earlier, Amino et al. sought to show that the performance of the FT4 test in pregnancy was strongly affected by residual albumin interference [26]. This was refuted by a paper showing that in late pregnancy, albumin and FT4 levels both fell significantly, giving a strong physiological correlation [46]. This relationship was falsely linked to a significant albumin-binding artefact. Additionally, many studies attempted to prove test invalidity by the results of addition of serum albumin in vitro [24, 25]. A paper describing the effects of various sources and purities of albumin showed a notable phenomenon that explained the apparent severity of the albumin effect. Namely, purified albumin in vitro has very variable and often much stronger binding characteristics compared with albumin in vivo, thereby grossly exaggerating the perceived problem [24, 28].

The second criticism emanated from the Ekins's laboratory. Here it was alleged that the then available analogue assays should not work in the conditions described. This argument persisted for almost 20 years before dying away in the face of contradictory evidence. Simply put, Ekins's analysis and equations pertained only to the ambient FT4 concentration. It did not take into account the working of the practical assay, where FT4 was measured by the T4 actually bound on to an antibody probe and calibrated in FT4 units [47–50]. This could amount to 150–200 times the ambient FT4, thereby diluting Ekins's alleged interferences by this factor [51]. Note: a free hormone assay is valid so long as the measuring system does not significantly affect the bound/free equilibrium of the hormone in serum.

The third criticism was from the Nelson group [52–55]. This group, in their analysis, made a fundamental mistake in their studies. Of all the assays in the biochemical field, FT4 and FT3 assays are unique in the limited ways they can be legitimately studied. In short, the reactants in free hormone assays work together like a clock. It is not possible to separate individual aspects of the test and study them independently, and the tests typical of validation of a total analyte do not apply. Their allegations amounted to a complaint that individual pieces of the mechanism did not reflect the whole test's actual performance. Thereby, the whole of this work can be dismissed as basically unsound [56].

The fourth criticism emanated from the Soldin group [57–60]. This group attempted to show that mass spectrometry and ultrafiltration give results superior in their accuracy to immunoassays. Unfortunately, in the period in which their results led to this claim, their test method was performed at 25 °C [61]. It is known that assays for FT4/3 must be performed at 37 °C. This is because the binding properties of TBG change differently from those of transthyretin and albumin at unphysiological temperatures [62–64]. The likelihood of artefacts appears especially in the paper of Gu et al. [58], where, as well as invalidated by the wrong temperature conditions, the resulting reference range for FT3 was artificially extremely wide, owing possibly to a larger Donnan effect on the more weakly bound analyte [65]. No valid assay method can depict the FT3 reference range as being wider than that of total T3 [59]. No papers, including this, issued before 2010 can therefore be valid. It gives me no pleasure to find that, in later papers presumably using the correct higher temperature, supporting reference is made with these earlier spurious assertions. This does not seem to be solid science and, by acting in this way, discredits later communications.

9.5 Recommendations for the Future

It is now clear that FT4 and FT3 assays are in urgent need of rationalising between manufacturers [66–72]. This comes about because of the more refined measurements that are needed for their new-found greater importance in diagnosis. I have already written on this subject, in which regulators, manufacturers and users are criticised for their collective failure in adequately addressing the problem [73]. Lack of harmonisation also can have an additional confounding effect in meta-analytic studies, where the results from different manufacturers' tests have been amalgamated. The problem adds an extra unwanted complication to the validity of such work and indeed any that have been subjected to different assays in the course of a particular investigation.

If persuasion has not succeeded, then it becomes the responsibility of regulators to demand that all assays must obey certain essential rules if they are to be permitted to market. These indispensable rules are (a) FT4, and to a certain extent FT3, assays must be robust to serial dilution (i.e. maintaining close to constant values), (b) correlating with a "gold standard" equilibrium method with a slope and correlation close to unity and an extrapolation close to the origin [73]. A parallel viewpoint can be obtained by plotting FT4, using the factor (FT4, equilibrium dialysis-FT4 test) against serum dilution, termed the serum-binding capacity (sBC) [74]. In this case, a valid assay should show only a small negative gradient with serum dilution. Not many assays obey these rules. One that does so is the Vitros eCi method [75–77]. These papers comparing commercial assays show significant differences in performance [76, 77]. Nor can we assume that calibration over the range is strictly proportional. Papers merely comparing one commercial assay against another fail to consider that both may be in error compared with equilibrium dialysis.

Given the existence of methods that obey rules for valid FT4 and FT3 assays, it is rather strange that these tests figure so little in the literature. The reason may well lie in the separation of purchase and use. Assays are now platform-driven and must be bought and used as such. If the buyer has little knowledge of the purchase, and the user is indifferent, it is too easy to believe that financial inducement then trumps quality. In many ways, the sale of all-in platforms tends to lock the user in even though some may offer tests of poorer quality, but the user is locked in. In former times, users could have much wider choices and freedom to purchase than is the case today.

Finally, it is rather depressing but inevitable that poorer FT4 and FT3 assays are widely criticised and, as shown earlier in including better assays in a general denunciation, have lamentably encouraged false beliefs now embedded in the literature (see the dissection of fallacies above). It is striking that few papers describing the use of the Vitros method appear in publications and where they do, criticisms are muted. Perhaps it is a truth in this field, as in others, that product insufficiency invites more comment than adequacy. However, in view of this refutation of the criticisms, it is to be hoped that they will now cease.

9.6 A New Paradigm for Diagnosis and Treatment?

The now-realised central importance of FT4 and FT3 measurements in diagnosis and treatment of hypothyroid patients invites a consideration of an improved paradigm to aid optimal treatment. The FT3 to FT4 ratio is an approximate indication of combined thyroidal production of T3 and corporeal T4/T3 conversion. In health, this ratio describes the balance point unique to the individual and, if archived to monitor future problems, can provide serum FT3/FT4 values to give a guideline for suitable later treatment. Additionally, the individual FT4 and FT3 concentrations give an indication of the patient's conversion capabilities within the respective ranges. Further, if a patient presents as unwell, it may be possible to differentiate illness of a non-thyroidal and thyroid deficiency per se. The FT3 to FT4 ratio should be lower in the range, owing to inhibition of T4-T3 conversion. Conversely, with thyroid dysfunction, the ratio will be higher, owing to the effects of loss of T4 production by the thyroid, with compensated maintenance of T3 production through feed-forward protection by the diseased gland itself. This concept, though requiring a significant re-evaluation of the importance of FT3, can be easily researched in a long-term project.

9.7 Conclusion

This review demonstrates the urgent need for re-evaluation and redesign of FT4 and FT3 assays, now that their central importance in diagnosis and treatment is becoming clear. It is, however, perplexing that tests obeying the definitive requirements of valid assays exist, but yet find relatively little evidence of use in the literature. It can only be concluded that users of the tests have little liaison with purchasers, being indifferent to what is being bought. If biochemical tests are to be used, it is surely necessary to have ongoing confidence in the accuracy of the results over the whole assay spectrum and with many different patient groups. Additionally, it is clear, from the invalid criticisms of FT4 and FT3 one-step assays and attempts to develop assays that work at room temperature, that users seem to have little or no grasp of the physical chemistry that lies behind their operation. In this regard, the lacuna between medical practice and lack of attention to the quality of the tests used has significantly hindered progress and has coarsened the outcome of research, especially in meta-analyses. Recommendations for harmonisation have long been proposed, with little discernible improvement. If users and manufacturers will not act, the responsibility now lies firmly at the regulators' door to forcibly rectify the situation, by applying the appropriate requirements for use. Nonetheless, the mechanistic thinking typical of thyroid diagnosis today needs reassessment in the light of new knowledge revisiting the working of the HPT axis. Patients deserve no less.

References

1. Murray GR. Note on the treatment of myxoedema by hypodermic injections of an extract of the thyroid gland of a sheep. Br Med J. 1891;10:796–7. https://doi.org/10.1136/bmj.2.1606.796.
2. Burgess AM. Myxoedema, controlled by thyroid extract for 52 years: case. Ann Intern Med. 1946;25:146–50.
3. Harington CR, Barger G. Chemistry of thyroxine constitution and synthesis of thyroxine. Biochem J. 1927;21(1):169–83.
4. Gross J, Pitt-Rivers R. 3:5:3′-Triiodothyronine. 1. Isolation from thyroid gland and synthesis. Biochem J. 1953;53:645–52. https://doi.org/10.1042/bj0530645.
5. Hennessey JV. Historical and current perspective in the use of thyroid extracts for the treatment of hypothyroidism. Endocr Pract. 2015;21:1161–70. https://doi.org/10.4158/EP14477.RA.
6. McAninch EA, Bianco AC. The history and future of treatment of hypothyroidism. Ann Intern Med. 2016;164:50–6. https://doi.org/10.7326/M15-1799.

7. Murphy BEP, Pattee CJ, Gold A. Clinical evaluation of a new method for the determination of serum thyroxine. J Clin Endocrinol. 1966;26:245–56. https://doi.org/10.1210/jcem2-6-23-247.
8. Acland JD. The interpretation of the serum protein-bound iodine: a review. J Clin Pathol. 1971;24:187–218. https://doi.org/10.1136/jcp.24.3.187.
9. Neild JE, Byfield PGH, Lalloz MRA, Tait D, Marigold JH, Croft DN, Slavin BM. Familial abnormalities of thyroxine-binding proteins: some problems of recognition and interpretation. J Clin Pathol. 1985;38:327–30. https://doi.org/10.1136/jcp.38.3.327.
10. Ekins RP, Williams ES, Ellis S. The sensitive and precise measurement of serum thyroxine by saturation analysis (competitive protein-binding assay). Clin Biochem. 1969;2:253–88. https://doi.org/10.1016/S0009-9120(68)80083-9.
11. Woldring MG, Bakker A, Doorenbos H. In vitro uptake of radioactive 131I-labelled L-triiodothyronine by human erythrocytes as an index of thyroid function. Eur J Endocrinol. 1960;34:305–11. https://doi.org/10.1530/acta.0.XXXIV0305.
12. Lee RH, Spencer CA, Mestman JH, Miller EA, Petrovic I, Braverman LE, Goodwin TM. Free T4 immunoassays are flawed in pregnancy. Am J Obstet Gynecol. 2009;200(260):e1–260. https://doi.org/10.1016/j.ajog.2008.10.042.
13. Midgley JEM. Thyroid hormone-uptake test: a concept based on false premises. J Clin Ligand Assay. 2006;29:146–51.
14. Midgley JEM, Christofides ND. Free thyroxine assays: no going back. Am J Obstet Gynecol. 2009;202:e6. https://doi.org/10.1016/j.ajog.2009.08.033.
15. Jansen HI, van Herwaarden AE, Huijgen HJ, Painter RC, Hillebrand JJ, Boelen A, Heijboer AC. Pregnancy disrupts the accuracy of automated fT4 immunoassays. Eur Thyroid J. 2022;11:e220145. https://doi.org/10.1530/ETJ-22-0145.
16. Larsen PR, Dockalova J, Sipula D, Wu FM. Immunoassay of thyroxine in unextracted human serum. J Clin Endocrinol Metab. 1973;37:177–82. https://doi.org/10.1210/jcem-37-2-177.
17. Hesch RD, Evered DC. Radioimmunoassay of triiodothyronine in unextracted human serum. Br Med J. 1973;1:645–8. https://doi.org/10.1136/jcp.29.12.1054.
18. Utiger RD. Radioimmunoassay of human plasma thyrotropin*. J Clin Invest. 1965;44:1277–86. https://doi.org/10.1172/JCI105234.
19. Spencer CA. Laboratory thyroid tests: a historical perspective. Thyroid. 2023;33:407–19. https://doi.org/10.1089/thy.2022.0397.
20. Ekins RP. Methods for the measurement of free thyroid hormones. In: Free thyroid hormones, Int Symposium, Venice. 1979;479:72–92. ISBN 0444901051, 9780444901057.
21. Midgley JEM, Wilkins TA. New methods of free thyroid hormone assay. In: Bizollon CA, editor. Physiological peptides and new trends in radioimmunoassay. Amsterdam: Elsevier; 1981. p. 215–34. ISBN 0-444-80358-0.
22. Wilkins TA, Midgley JEM, Barron N. Comprehensive study of a thyroxin-analog-based assay for free thyroxin ("AmerlexFT4"). Clin Chem. 1985;31:1644–53. https://doi.org/10.1093/clinchem/31.10.1644.
23. Midgley JEM, Moon CR, Wilkins TA. Validity of analog free thyroxin immunoassays. Part II. Clin Chem. 1987;33:2145–52. https://doi.org/10.1093/clinchem/33.12.2145.
24. Bayer MF. Free thyroxine results are affected by albumin concentration and nonthyroidal illness. Clin Chim Acta. 1983;130:391–6. https://doi.org/10.1016/0009-8981(83)90315-7.
25. Stockigt JR, Stevens V, White EL, Barlow JW. "Unbound analog" radioimmunoassays for free thyroxin measure the albumin-bound hormone fraction. Clin Chem. 1983;29:1408–10. https://doi.org/10.1093/clinchem/29.7.1408.
26. Amino N, Nishi K, Nakatani K, Mizuta H, Ichihara K, et al. Effect of albumin concentration on the assay of serum free thyroxin by equilibrium radioimmunoassay with labeled thyroxin analog (Amerlex Free T4). Clin Chem. 1983;29:321–5. https://doi.org/10.1093/clinchem/29.2.321.
27. Lee WN, Golden MP, Van Herle AJ, Lippe BM, Kaplan SA. Inherited abnormal thyroid hormone-binding protein causing selective increase of total serum thyroxine. J Clin Endocrinol Metab. 1979;49:292–9. https://doi.org/10.1210/jcem-49-2-292.

28. Hashimoto T, Matsubara F. A comment on the "albumin effect" in analog free-thyroxin determinations. Clin Chem. 1987;33:1291–3. https://doi.org/10.1093/clinchem/33.7.1291a.
29. Chatzitomaris A, Hoermann R, Midgley JEM, Hering S, Urban A, Dietrich B, Abood A, Klein HH, Dietrich JW. Thyroid allostasis-adaptive responses of thyrotropic feedback control to conditions of strain, stress, and developmental programming. Front Endocrinol (Lausanne). 2017;8:163. https://doi.org/10.3389/fendo.2017.00163.
30. Allan DJ, Murphy F, Needham CF, Wilkins TA, Barron N, Midgley JE. Sensitive test for thyroid hormone autoantibodies in serum. Lancet. 1982;2(8302):824. https://doi.org/10.1016/S0140-6736(82)92716-7.
31. Christofides ND, Sheehan CP, Midgley JEM. One-step, labeled-antibody assay for measuring free thyroxin. I. Assay development and validation. Clin Chem. 1992;38:11–8. https://doi.org/10.1093/clinchem/38.1.11.
32. Sheehan CP, Christofides ND. One-step, labeled-antibody assay for measuring free thyroxin. II. Performance in a multicentre trial. Clin Chem. 1992;38:19–25. https://doi.org/10.1093/clinchem/38.1.19.
33. Christofides ND, Sheehan CP. Enhanced chemiluminescence labeled-antibody immunoassay (Amerlite-MAB) for free thyroxine: design, development, and technical validation. Clin Chem. 1995;41:17–23. https://doi.org/10.1093/clinchem/41.1.17.
34. Christofides ND, Sheehan CP. Multicenter evaluation of enhanced chemiluminescence labeled-antibody. Immunoassay (Amerlite-MAB) for free thyroxine. Clin Chem. 1995;41:24–31. https://doi.org/10.1093/clinchem/41.1.24.
35. Ursem SR, Boelen A, Hillebrand JJ, den Elzen WPJ, Annemieke C, Heijboer AC. How low can we (reliably) go? A method comparison of TSH assays with a focus on low concentrations. Eur Thyroid J. 2023;12:e230123. https://doi.org/10.1530/ETJ-23-0123.
36. Sheehan MT. Biochemical testing of the thyroid: TSH is the best and, oftentimes, only test needed—a review for primary care. Clin Med Res. 2016;14:83–92. https://doi.org/10.3121/cmr.2016.1309.
37. Spencer CA, LoPresti JS, Patel A, Guttler RB, et al. Applications of a new chemiluminometric thyrotropin assay to subnormal measurement. J Clin Endocrinol Metab. 1990;70:453. https://doi.org/10.1210/jcem-70-2-453.
38. Hamilton TE, Davis S, Onstad L, Kopecky KJ. Thyrotropin levels in a population with no clinical, autoantibody, or ultrasonographic evidence of thyroid disease: implications for the diagnosis of subclinical hypothyroidism. J Clin Endocrinol Metab. 2008;93:1224–30. https://doi.org/10.1210/jc.2006-2300.
39. Hoermann R, Midgley JEM. TSH measurement and its implications for personalised clinical decision-making. J Thyroid Res. 2012;2012:438037. https://doi.org/10.1155/2012/438037.
40. Rothacker KM, Brown SJ, Hadlow NC, Wardrop R, Walsh JP. Reconciling the log-linear and non–log-linear nature of the TSH-free T4 relationship: intra-individual analysis of a large population. J Clin Endocrinol Metab. 2016;101:151–8. https://doi.org/10.1210/jc.2015-4011.
41. Chu JW, Crapo LM. The treatment of subclinical hypothyroidism is seldom necessary (Review). J Clin Endocrinol Metab. 2001;86:4591–9. https://doi.org/10.1210/jcem.86.10.796.1.
42. Calissendorff J, Falhammar H. To treat or not to treat subclinical hypothyroidism, what is the evidence? Medicina (Kaunas). 2020;56:40. https://doi.org/10.3390/medicina56010040.
43. Hoermann R, Midgley JEM, Larisch R, Dietrich JW. Integration of peripheral and glandular regulation of triiodothyronine production by thyrotropin in untreated and thyroxine-treated subjects. Horm Metab Res. 2015;47:674–80. https://doi.org/10.1055/s-0034-1398616.
44. Hoermann R, Midgley JEM, Larisch R, Dietrich JW. Recent advances in thyroid hormone regulation: toward a new paradigm for optimal diagnosis and treatment. Front Endocrinol (Lausanne). 2017;8:364. https://doi.org/10.3389/fendo.2017.00364.
45. Hoermann R, Pekker M, Midgley JEM, Larisch R, Dietrich JW. Principles of endocrine regulation: reconciling tensions between robustness in performance and adaptation to change. Front Endocrinol (Lausanne). 2022;13:825107. https://doi.org/10.3389/fendo.2022.825107.

46. Ball R, Freedman DB, Holmes CR, Midgley JEM, Sheehan CP. Low-normal concentrations of free thyroxin in serum in late pregnancy: physiological fact, not technical artefact. Clin Chem. 1989;35:1891–6. https://doi.org/10.1093/clinchem/35.9.1891.
47. Ekins RP, Jackson TM, Edwards P. More on the Amerlex kit analog method for thyroxin. Clin Chem. 1986;32:1243–6. https://doi.org/10.1093/clinchem/32.6.
48. Elkins R. Measurement of free hormones in blood (review). Endocr Rev. 1990;11:5–46. https://doi.org/10.1210/edrv-11-1-5.
49. Ekins R. The free hormone hypothesis and measurement of free hormones. Clin Chem. 1992;38:1289–93. https://doi.org/10.1093/clinchem/38.7.1289.
50. Ekins R. Analytic measurements of free thyroxine. Clin Lab Med. 1993;13:599–630. https://doi.org/10.1016/S0272-2712(18)30428-1.
51. Midgley JEM. The design of one-step free thyroxine assays: a critique. J Clin Ligand Assay. 2005;28:110–5.
52. Nelson JC, Nayak SS, Wilcox RB. Variable underestimates by serum free thyroxine (T4) immunoassays of free T4 concentrations in simple solutions. J Clin Endocrinol Metab. 1994;79:1373–5. https://doi.org/10.1210/jcem.79.5.7962331.
53. Wang R, Nelson JC, Weiss RM, Wilcox RB. Accuracy of free thyroxine measurements across natural ranges of thyroxine binding to serum proteins. Thyroid. 2000;10:31–9. https://doi.org/10.1089/thy.2000.10.31.
54. Nelson JC, Wang R, Asher DT, Wilcox RB. The nature of analogue-based free thyroxine estimates. Thyroid. 2004;14:1030–6. https://doi.org/10.1089/thy.2004.14.1030.
55. Fritz K, Wilcox RB, Nelson JC. A direct free thyroxine (T4) immunoassay with the characteristics of a total T4 immunoassay. Clin Chem. 2007;53:911–5. https://doi.org/10.1373/clinchem.2006.083915.
56. Midgley JEM, Christofides ND. Legitimate and illegitimate tests of free-analyte assay function. Clin Chem. 2009;55:439–41. https://doi.org/10.1373/clinchem.2008.116525.
57. Soldin OP, ,Tractenberg RE, Hollowell JG, Jonklaas J, Janicic N, Soldin SJ. Trimester-specific changes in maternal thyroid hormone, thyrotropin, and thyroglobulin concentrations during gestation: trends and associations across trimesters in iodine sufficiency. Thyroid 2004;14:1084–1090. doi: https://doi.org/10.1089/thy.2004.14.1084.
58. Soldin SJ, Soukhova N, Janicic N, Jonklass J, Soldin OP. The measurement of free thyroxine by isotope dilution tandem mass spectrometry. Clin Chim Acta. 2005;358:113–8. https://doi.org/10.1016/j.cccn.2005.02.010.
59. Gu J, Soldin OP, Steven J, Soldin SJ. Simultaneous quantification of free triiodothyronine and free thyroxine by isotope dilution tandem mass spectrometry. Clin Biochem. 2007;40:1386–91. https://doi.org/10.1016/j.clinbiochem.2007.08.007.
60. Kahric-Janicic N, Soldin SJ, Soldin OP, West T, Gu J, Jonklaas J. Tandem mass spectrometry improves the accuracy of free thyroxine measurements during pregnancy. Thyroid. 2007;17:303–11. https://doi.org/10.1089/thy.2006.0303.
61. Christofides ND, Midgley JEM. Inaccuracies in free thyroid hormone measurement by ultrafiltration and tandem mass spectrometry. Clin Chem. 2009;55:2228–9. https://doi.org/10.1373/clinchem.2009.134593.
62. Ross HA, Benraad TJ. Is free thyroxine accurately measurable at room temperature? Clin Chem. 1992;38:880–6. https://doi.org/10.1093/clinchem/38.6.880.
63. van der Sluis Veer G, Vermes I, Bonte HA, Hoorn RKJ. Temperature effects on free-thyroxine measurements: analytical and clinical consequences. Clin Chem. 1992;38:1327–31. https://doi.org/10.1093/clinchem/38.7.1327.
64. Qi X, Chan WL, Read RJ, Zhou A, Carrell RW. Temperature-responsive release of thyroxine and environmental adaptation in Australians. Proc Biol Sci. 2014;281:20132747. https://doi.org/10.1098/rspb.2013.2747.
65. Donnan FG. Theorie der Membrangleichgewichte und Membranpotentiale bei Vorhandensein von nicht dialysierenden Elektrolyten. Ein Beitrag zur physikalisch-chemischen Physiologie (Theory of membrane equilibria and membrane potentials in the presence of non-dialyzing

electrolytes. A contribution to physical-chemical physiology). Z Elektrochem Angew Phys Chem. 1911;17:572–81.
66. Midgley JEM. "All that glisters is not gold": ultrafiltration and free thyroxine measurement. With apologies to W Shakespeare. Clin Biochem. 2010;44:151–3. https://doi.org/10.1016/j.clinbiochem.2010.11.001.
67. Thienpont LM, Beastall G, Christofides ND, Faix JD, Ieiri T, Jarrige V, Miller WG, Miller R, Nelson JC, Ronin C, Ross HA, Rottmann M, Thijssen JH, Toussaint B. Scientific Division Working Group for Standardization of Thyroid Function Tests (WG-STFT): proposal of a candidate international conventional reference measurement procedure for free thyroxine in serum. Clin Chem Lab Med. 2007;45:934–6. https://doi.org/10.1515/CCLM.2007.155.
68. Thienpont LM, Van Uytfanghe K, Beastall G, Faix JD, Ieiri T, Miller WG, Nelson JC, Ronin C, Ross HA, Thijssen JH, Toussaint B. Report of the IFCC Working Group for Standardization of Thyroid Function Tests; part 2: free thyroxine and free triiodothyronine. Clin Chem. 2010;56:912–20. https://doi.org/10.1373/clinchem.2009.140194.
69. Thienpont LM, Faix JD, Beastall G. Standardisation of free T4 and harmonization of TSH measurements. A request for input from endocrinologists and other physicians. Eur Thyroid J. 2015;4:271–2. https://doi.org/10.1159/000440614.
70. IFCC. Standardization of thyroid function tests. Available from http://www.ifcc.org/ifcc-scientific-division/sd-committees/c-stft/
71. Kratzsch J, Baumann NA, Ceriotti F, et al. Global FT4 immunoassay standardization: an expert opinion review. Clin Chem Lab Med. 2021;59:1013–23. https://doi.org/10.1515/cclm-2020-1696.
72. Sapin R, Gasser F, Blicklé J-F. Dosages de thyroxine libre: une harmonisation plus que jamais necessaire. Free thyroxine immunoassays: harmonization is more than ever required. Presse Med. 2008;37:1189–91. https://doi.org/10.1016/j.lpm.2008.03.005.
73. Midgley JEM, et al. Global FT4 immunoassay standardization: an expert opinion review. Clin Chem Lab Med. 2021;59:e223–4. https://doi.org/10.1515/cclm-2021-0036.
74. Midgley JEM, Christofides ND. Rationalizing free thyroid hormone assay performance. J Clin Ligand Assay. 2008;31:55–6.
75. Christofides ND, Wilkinsn E, Stoddart M, Dc R, Beckett GJ. Serum thyroxine binding capacity-dependent bias in an automated free thyroxine assay. J Immunoass. 1999;20:201–21. https://doi.org/10.1080/01971529909349351.
76. Christofides ND, Wilkinson E, Stoddart M, Ray DC, Beckett GJ. Assessment of serum thyroxine binding capacity-dependent biases in free thyroxine assays. Clin Chem. 1999;45:520–5. https://doi.org/10.1093/CLINCHEM/45.4.520.
77. Sapin R. Serum thyroxine binding capacity-dependent bias in five free thyroxine immunoassays: assessment with serum dilution experiments and impact on diagnostic performance. Clin Biochem. 2001;34:367–71. https://doi.org/10.1016/s0009-9120(01)00241-7.

Chapter 10
Diagnosis of Hypothyroidism

Rudolf Hoermann and Johannes W. Dietrich

10.1 Diagnostic Considerations

Clinical diagnosis is readily possible when the typical aspects of the phenotype of hypothyroidism are present in the full manifestation of the syndrome (Sect. 7.1). *Leading signs* are, among others, a slowdown of physical and mental functions, fatigue, weight gain, cold intolerance, dry and pale skin, scrubby hair, bloated face, eyelid oedema, bradycardia and hyporeflexia. The diagnostic value of these symptoms lies more in their *combined expression*, because many of them are subtle or non-specific when viewed in isolation. The fully developed syndrome is however already often a sign of a long history of patient suffering. In extremis, a life-threatening exacerbation of *myxedematous coma* may occur, facilitated by an unrecognised disease and precipitated by other stressful events.

R. Hoermann (✉)
Yandina, QLD, Australia

Department of General Internal Medicine, Gastroenterology and Endocrinology, [Retired] Klinikum Lüdenscheid, Lüdenscheid, Germany
e-mail: rudolf.hoermann@gmail.com

J. W. Dietrich
Diabetes, Endocrinology and Metabolism Section, Department of Medicine, St. Josef-Hospital, Ruhr University Hospitals, Bochum, Germany

Centre for Diabetes Technology (ZDT), Catholic Hospitals Bochum, Bochum, Germany

Centre for Rare Endocrine Diseases (ZSEK), Ruhr Center for Rare Diseases (CeSER), Ruhr University of Bochum and Witten/Herdecke University, Bochum, Germany

Centre for Thyroid Medicine (ZSM), Ruhr University of Bochum, Bochum, Germany
e-mail: johannes.dietrich@ruhr-uni-bochum.de

R. Hoermann, J. W. Dietrich (eds.), *Hypothyroidism*,
https://doi.org/10.1007/978-981-96-3682-2_10

Hypothyroid *symptom scoring* has been suggested by some authors, but a lack of sensitivity and specificity has not supported their recommendation in routine clinical application [1, 2]. More recently more specific questionnaires have been designed and validated to assess thyroid-related complaints and other quality of life impairments in hypothyroid patients (Sect. 7.9).

Oligosymptomatic manifestations and more subtle symptoms of hypothyroidism are however much more prevalent. Variable symptoms and complaints may arise from the profound physiological effects of thyroid hormones on many organs, including the cardiovascular system, gastrointestinal tract, musculoskeletal system, fat, central and peripheral neurological system, mental health and metabolic consequences. As the hypothyroid symptoms *overlap* with numerous non-specific complaints and other diseases, considering the possibility of the presence of hypothyroidism may often be a first step towards the right diagnosis, seeking further direction and confirmation with extended biochemical testing and ultrasonographic imaging of the thyroid gland.

The diagnosis of *autoimmune thyroid disease* can be made with the detection of its typical marker, thyroid peroxidase (TPO) antibodies, in elevated concentrations. This may provide an important clue to the possible diagnosis of hypothyroidism, as does a characteristic ultrasonographic appearance of the gland. However, the detection of an immunological marker is not synonymous with the presence of the functional disease of hypothyroidism, because autoimmune thyroiditis at an early stage is frequently *associated with euthyroidism*, and Graves' disease may be in functional remission with the immunological marker still present.

If evidence for thyroid autoimmunity is present, testing is warranted for *other autoimmune disorders* that are associated with autoimmune thyroiditis and hypothyroidism [3]. This is most relevant for Addison's disease, termed Schmidt's syndrome in coexistence with Hashimoto's disease. We note that any cortisol deficiency (hypocortisolism) must be corrected prior to treating hypothyroidism with thyroid hormones to avoid a potentially life-threatening exacerbation of pre-existing Addison's disease (Addisonian crisis) [4]. Cortisol deficiency may also be associated with secondary hypothyroidism when pituitary disease is the cause of secondary hypothyroidism [5]. Both conditions must then be corrected concomitantly.

With the availability of highly sensitive methods for measuring thyroid-stimulating hormone (TSH), clinicians have increasingly given a key role to biochemical testing in the diagnosis of hypothyroidism, irrespective of the presence of hypothyroid symptoms [6]. Unlike any other indirect measure of organ function in endocrinology, the pituitary hormone TSH has thereby been given a special status and a pre-eminent position in defining primary hypothyroidism. For convenience, a new disease class of *subclinical hypothyroidism* in asymptomatic patients has been introduced, based solely on the presence of an elevated TSH concentration while the thyroid hormones FT3 and FT4 remain within their respective reference ranges [6]. The biochemical diagnosis of hypothyroidism defined as overt hypothyroidism requires, in addition to an elevated TSH, the presence of an FT4 concentration below its reference range.

The use of these relaxed definitions has elevated "hypothyroidism" to the most frequently diagnosed endocrine disease, affecting more than 10% of the population in Western countries (Sect. 1.2). Unfortunately, the clinically *important distinction* between hypothyroidism and subclinical hypothyroidism is frequently obscured in the literature, particularly in studies where TSH is used as the sole marker. The *threshold of TSH* when to recommend treatment is also a matter of uncertainty and ongoing debate.

10.1.1 Diagnostic Use of TSH

The current practice of a *TSH-centred* diagnostic approach to hypothyroidism invites important caveats because TSH has been increasingly recognised to be less reliable as a definitive diagnostic tool than previously assumed [7, 8] (Chap. 8). Recent advances in the understanding of the complex network of the hypothalamic–pituitary–thyroid axis regulation have led to a more differentiated view on the role of TSH, thereby denying its continued oversimplistic application in defining thyroid function in clinical medicine (Chap. 5). In a recent meta-analysis, thyroid hormones were found to be more closely correlated with patient symptomatology than with TSH [9]. Furthermore, owing to its nature as a controlling element rather than target in the complex network of hypothalamic–pituitary–thyroid axis regulation, the *univariate statistical derivation* of a TSH reference range is inherently ill-defined [10–12]. Even in the univariate case, the reference interval is not universally agreed on or adjusted for various influences, such as ethnicity, age and iodine supply [13–18].

Major shortcoming and errors in TSH testing, discussed in detail earlier, are summarised in Table 10.1.

Table 10.1 Issues with TSH testing

Diagnostic *ambiguity* of a given TSH value frequently arises for various reasons.
TSH is *controlling* by design, as opposed to being reflective of the peripheral thyroid state.
Different *aetiologies* that lead to TSH elevation result in statistical conflation when aggregated.
TSH shows a high *individuality and clustering effect* in its joined expressions with thyroid hormones.
TSH measurement is prone to *statistical fallacies* resulting from the use of population statistics for highly individual parameters.
The existence of pituitary–thyroid *linkage* of the TSH and FT4 (FT3) curves and their distribution in a population deny accuracy of univariate considerations.

10.1.2 TSH Reference Range

The *reference range* of TSH is statistically defined as the 95% confidence interval of a sufficiently large sample of healthy subjects drawn from the population. Adjusting for additional influences such as age, gender, body mass, iodine deficiency and pregnancy is a minor issue [19, 20]. Greater issues of interpretability arise from the fact that TSH and FT4 are interlocked, as the latter is raised to the healthy level by the former. TSH-FT4 pairs are therefore *clustered* in the population, defining a balance point (personal working point) between them [7, 12, 21] (Chap. 5). Consequently, variations for both the controlling and controlled hormone within a subject, are kept in a *narrow range*, compared to the wider (twice as wide as in an individual) range in the population, which depends on between-subject variation [22].

Three TSH ranges of interest are illustrated in Fig. 10.1, i.e. the *reference range* of a population, *normal range* of an individual and the *personal working point* (also known as the personal set point). Their width in a population decreases in that order [23].

This may explain why merely bringing the biochemistry within the accepted reference range may *not suffice* for patients to achieve their own healthy optimum that is required for symptom relief.

In the biochemical and symptomatic responses to LT4 treatment, the presence of the multileveled response groups and the intra-individual clustering effects have to be statistically accounted for and clinically considered (Fig. 10.2) [24]. Unmasking individual differences in the averaged treatment response uncovers clinically distinguishable subgroups within an indiscriminate patient panel. This forms the basis for

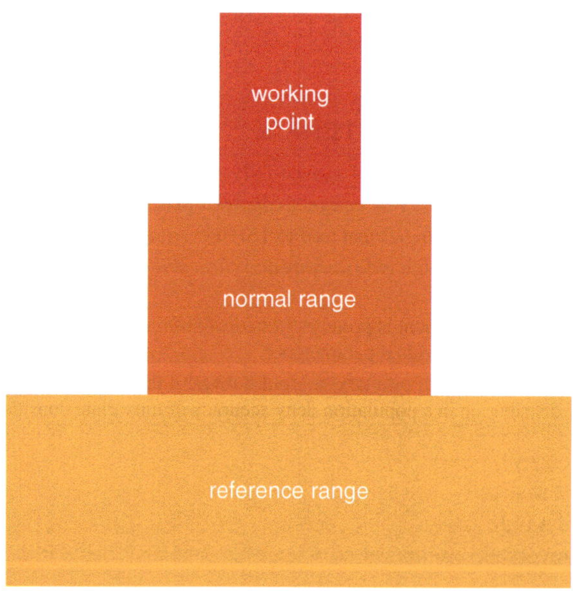

Fig. 10.1 Range considerations in the diagnostic use of TSH The reference range of a population is approximately twice as wide, compared to the normal range of an individual. The personal working point is even narrower at a given time. The normal range and working point vary by person and condition, moving within the population's range

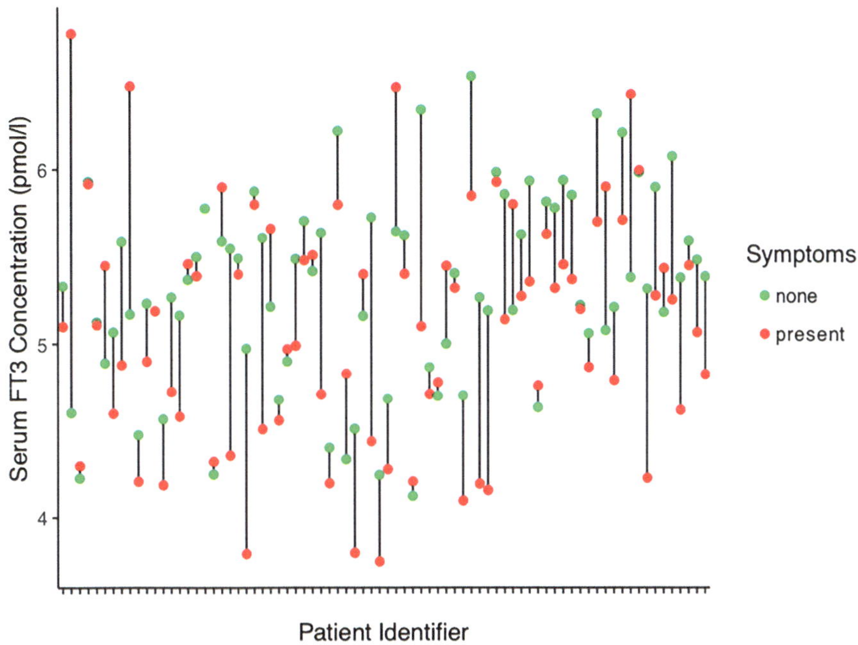

Fig. 10.2 Comparison of serum FT3 concentrations obtained from individual patients treated with levothyroxine after total thyroidectomy ($n = 77$) at two different occasions, (1) when complaining about hypothyroid symptoms, and (2) when asymptomatic after adjusting the LT4 dose. As can be seen, symptoms are associated with FT3 levels but not defined by an absolute FT3 position. A point refers to the average of either multiple symptomatic (red) or asymptomatic (green) presentations of a single patient during follow-up. (Data and figure are modified from Hoermann et al. [24])

the requirement to individualise the treatment of patients with hypothyroidism [23]. Range consideration alone is insufficient. Indeed, LT4 treatment can still be inefficient, potentially leaving the patient suffering from residual symptoms, when all three hormones, TSH, FT4 and FT3, are within their respective reference ranges. The reason being that each individual's situational working point and therapeutic window is narrow, and it is obscured by a much wider population range (Fig. 10.1) [24].

Furthermore, in the transition from the euthyroid to the hypothyroid state, the path of the *conditional balance point* in an individual contrasts with and separates from the cross-sectional TSH–FT4 relationship (Fig. 10.3) [23]. In a population, the strong correlation between logarithmic TSH and FT4 in the hypothyroid range disaggregates towards the euthyroid range, giving rise to several statistical phenomena, particularly stratification collider bias and *Simpson's paradox* [7, 25–30]. The property of *non-ergodicity* inherent to TSH and thyroid hormones introduces a bias to statistically averaged and correlative outcome studies [24]. This means that when data are analysed by cluster or person, correlations change, disappear or are even reversed, compared to the combined analysis of the data in the total group or

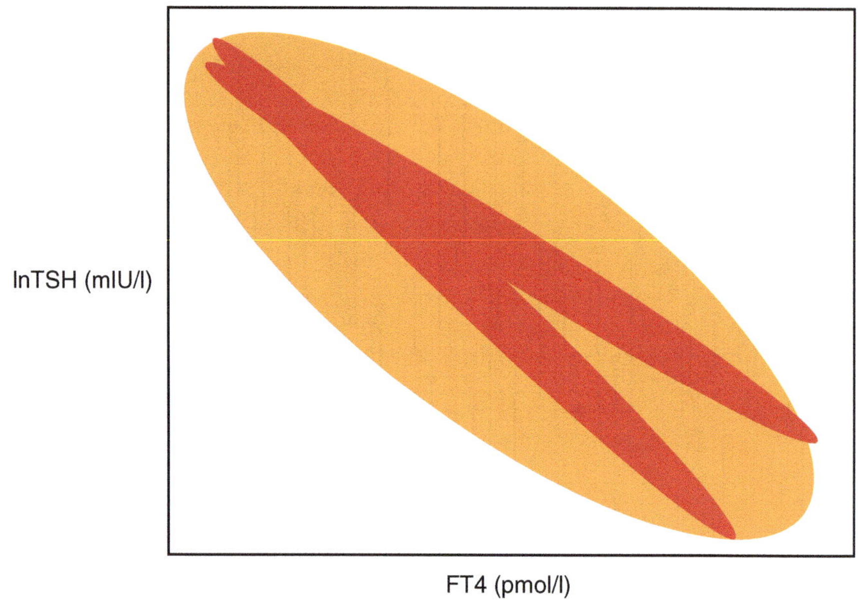

Fig. 10.3 Disaggregation of correlations between lnTSH and FT4 from the hypothyroid to euthyroid range between subjects
The trajectories of two individual patients, depicted by the red ellipses, do not follow the average relationship between lnTSH and FT4 in the population, surrounded by an orange ellipse. This behaviour gives rise to statistical aggregation bias (see text)

population [31–33]. The important clinical implication is a *lack of generalisation* of population-derived measures, such as thyroid function tests, thus demanding a personalised approach [23, 34].

Another issue is the assumption of an invariant log-linear gradient between TSH and FT4.

Traditionally, the relationship between TSH and FT4 in a population has been assumed to be *log-linear* over the total range [35–39]. However, this assumption proved to be more complex, with the relationship flattening in the euthyroid range [7, 25–30]. The gradient is rather *range-dependent*, displaying regional patterns of association unique to each of the different states of hypothyroidism, euthyroidism and hyperthyroidism [25, 28] (Fig. 10.4). Furthermore, gland mass interactions between the thyroid and pituitary glands are theoretically and physiologically inconsistent with the existence of a single logTSH gradient over the entire FT4 range, rather supporting a multi-regime relationship [30, 40] or hierarchical model with range-dependent *segmented relationships* [28].

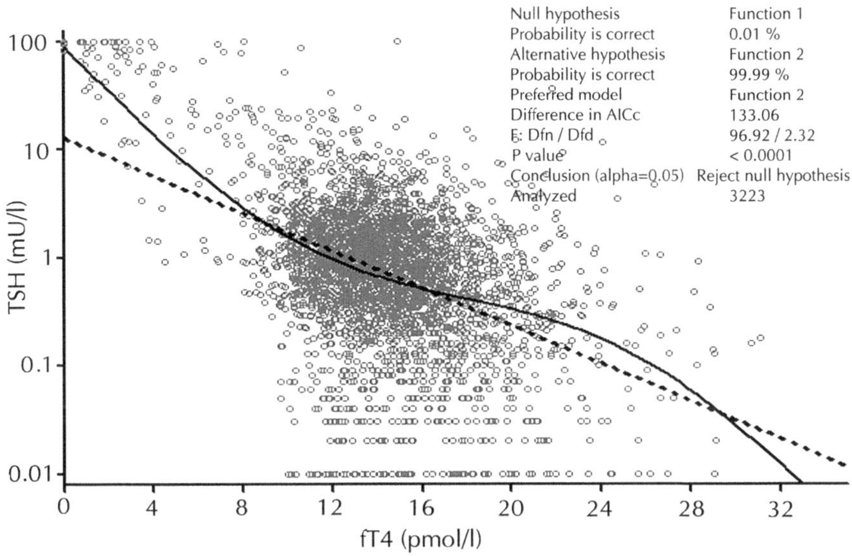

Fig. 10.4 Relationship between TSH and FT4 in a population
A straight line assuming a log-linear TSH–FT4 relationship (Function 1) does not statistically fit the data as well as a curvilinear relationship (Function 2), using Akaike's criteria (AIC). (Data and figure are from Hoermann et al. [25] and reproduced with permission of Oxford University Press)

As a consequence, the *diagnostic inaccuracy* of a TSH measurement inevitably increases when approaching the euthyroid range. The single simplistic TSH-centred method of defining the thyroid state *must fail* for that reason. It follows that a TSH measurement cannot be dissociated from both the clinical presentation of the patient and the thyroid hormones FT4 and FT3 nor from the specific underlying condition it applies to at a time. This is due to its intricate interlocking pattern with thyroid hormones, its personal trait-like property, non-ergodicity and statistical clustering effects [23, 24].

The *over-reliance on TSH* as a single biochemical test together with the absence of symptoms or non-specific nature of complaints raises an unsettling dilemma of diagnostic uncertainty [8]. Therefore, it is important to realise that in various diagnostic settings the role of TSH is different. This does require *separate consideration* of TSH measurement depending on whether it is used as a screening test, diagnostic tool or therapeutic target (Fig. 10.5).

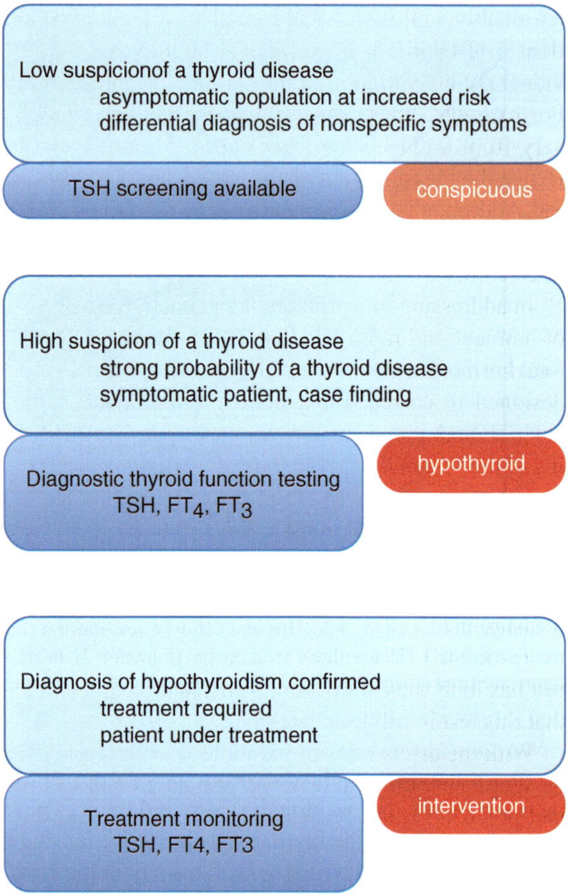

Fig. 10.5 Differential role of TSH in screening, diagnosis and treatment of hypothyroidism
The different roles cannot be unified, requiring differing cut-offs by context and support from the direct measurement of thyroid hormones (see text)

10.2 Clinical Use and Interpretation of Thyroid Parameters

Owing to its high sensitivity for primary thyroid failure, TSH qualifies as a suitable instrument for *screening* purposes, particularly in asymptomatic patients or patients with a possibility but low probability of hypothyroidism (Fig. 10.5). This provides an early indication to suggest a decline in thyroid hormone supply. In the case of an abnormal result, TSH measurement needs to be replaced by a more definitive testing including all three main thyroid hormones, FT4, FT3 and TSH. We also note that TSH testing must be repeated for confirmation so as not to rely on a single measurement. Due to the high individuality in the parameters, the limits of inferred "abnormality" should not necessarily be defined according to the population's reference range, rather being restricted to a narrower one, as explained above (Figs. 10.1, 10.2, 10.3 and 10.4). We tentatively suggest a TSH value outside a range between 0.6 and 2 mIU/l should encourage further testing, including the measurement of FT4 and FT3. A high value of TSH > 10 mIU/l greatly increases the likelihood of the presence of true hypothyroidism. This is mostly associated with a low FT4 concentration, with the latter then confirming the diagnosis of primary hypothyroidism.

In patients where leading *clinical symptoms* strongly suggest the diagnosis of hypothyroidism, the full test panel of TSH, FT4 and FT3 should be examined (Fig. 10.5). TSH testing alone will frequently fail, particularly since it does not address the possible diagnosis of secondary hypothyroidism, which is characterised by a low or normal TSH value, but low FT4 concentration. We also recommend that whenever there is an apparent conflict between the clinical aspect and biochemical test results, we must carefully consider the full panel of all three hormones and their interrelationships, thyroid imaging by ultrasound and measurements of other pituitary hormones. We note that not even that will rule out the diagnosis of hypothyroidism in rare conditions. Toxic chemicals being one example of a clinical manifestation of severe hypothyroidism in the presence of seemingly "normal" biochemical test results (Chap. 6.6.1).

The *diagnosis of primary hypothyroidism* can be unequivocally established by a combination of low FT4 concentrations and markedly elevated TSH levels [6]. The history, presentation and examination of the patient will uncover some symptomatology in most patients, even though they may not always be aware of them due to the long-standing disease.

Subclinical hypothyroidism is on the face of it an easy diagnosis, when going strictly by its guideline-based definition of a TSH concentration above the population's reference range and FT4 concentration still within its reference rage (6). However, the formal diagnosis as such does not imply a unique aetiological entity, the presence of clinical disease or a universal need of treatment of a patient with this laboratory constellation. The classification of subclinical hypothyroidism is generally *ill-defined* and not well placed and understood in the context of hypothalamic–pituitary–thyroid regulation [41] (Chap. 5). Due to the diagnostic ambiguity and remaining uncertainty, this diagnosis presents a dilemma for clinicians and patients alike [42]. Pertinent questions are not answered as to whether the many individuals, as many as 5–10% of the population, presenting with this prevalent constellation suffer from a true disease, and when this condition may require therapeutic intervention. This situation may be particularly difficult to accept for patients presenting with symptoms which are in their opinion suggestive of a thyroid condition [43, 44]. The apparent deficiencies of this approach and its lack of diagnostic specificity and reliability have been reviewed earlier. As explained there, the problem is fundamentally rooted in the principles of hypothalamus–pituitary–thyroid axis regulation [45]. Briefly, in patients with early thyroid failure due to autoimmune thyroiditis presenting with the laboratory constellation of subclinical hypothyroidism, compensatory action may successfully preserve FT3 homeostasis [11, 46]. The remaining functional thyroid tissue is then still able at this stage to support the enhanced feed-forward control of TSH and preferential T3 secretion, operative in the hypothalamic–pituitary–thyroid axis regulation. We note, as explained earlier, that the system is designed to take anticipatory and proactive action rather than reacting post hoc to a shortage of thyroid hormone supply to the body. The success or failure of the central attempt at compensation determines the onset of a clinical disease. A moderately elevated TSH concentration by itself cannot reliably discriminate between the two outcomes and remains therefore both ambiguous and diagnostically uncertain.

Apart from its diagnostic use, the laboratory constellation of subclinical hypothyroidism has been strongly implicated as a prognostic marker to increase the risk of, among other diseases, cardiovascular disease and mortality [47, 48]. Although the conclusion may hold true, this may be unrelated to and must be separated from thyroid failure and the early development of primary hypothyroidism [49, 50]. Rather the constellation of a slightly elevated TSH level together with "normal" thyroid hormone concentrations is shared by the prevalent *general stress response* of the body [49]. Working point adjustments of thyroid homeostasis occur in association with allostatic load type 2 including chronic psychosocial stress (Table 6.1). In this setting, such stressors increase the working point, so that TSH concentrations are also increased in the absence of hypothyroidism. *Stress* itself is, of course, a well-known and strong contributory factor to cardiovascular disease and mortality risk. *Genetic traits* further add to a high individual variability in the expression of the hypothalamic–pituitary–thyroid working point [51–55]. Differential associations of genetic footprints with FT3, FT4 and TSH have been reported to confer different risks [56]. Unfortunately, many prospective studies have *conflated* the entirely different mechanisms and clinical entities in performing statistically aggregated analyses over the different aetiologies, thereby obscuring the individual risk profiles [34].

When tested as a single parameter, for instance in thyroid disease screening, an elevated TSH value may arise from different conditions, which need to be *differentiated* by further testing (Fig. 10.5). Considerations in the differential diagnosis of a TSH elevation include a thyroid disease, TSH-producing pituitary tumour, the syndrome of reduced sensitivity to thyroid hormones, possible interferences with the measurement and transient situations such as the recovery phase of a low-T3 syndrome and other states of temporary imbalance between TSH and thyroid hormones (Table 7.2).

In summary, the diagnostic process of hypothyroidism includes a *synopsis* of clinical symptoms, morphological features (ultrasound) and complete biochemical testing including measurements of all three hormones FT3, FT4 and TSH, and, importantly, also consideration of their interrelations beyond statistical referencing. Particularly the *interdependence* and interaction between the hormones are of major interest according to the principles of thyroid homeostasis and relational stability (Chaps. 2 and 5). For instance, a combination of TSH and FT4 measurements suggests the disruption to the homeostatic balance in the case of secondary hypothyroidism due to hypopituitarism, presenting with a low FT4 level in the presence of a "normal" TSH level. Instead of the terms "reference" or "normal" based on univariate analysis of TSH and FT4, the term "appropriate" or "inappropriate" is suggested to express a joint evaluation. A synopsis of supportive and disrupted mechanisms in the hypothalamic–pituitary–thyroid axis regulation and their relevance for various forms of hypothyroidism is shown in Fig. 10.6.

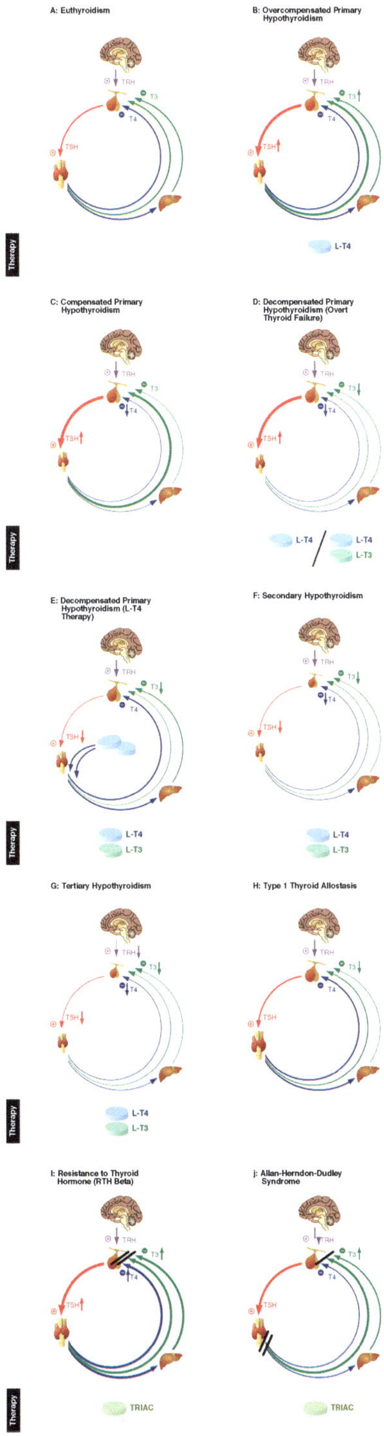

Fig. 10.6 Supportive and disruptive mechanisms in the hypothalamic–pituitary–thyroid axis regulations and their expression in various forms of hypothyroidism. A: Fully balanced state in euthyroidism; B: Overcompensation of incipient hypothyroidism by inappropriately elevated FT3 concentration; C: Fully compensated hypothyroidism with appropriately elevated FT3; D: Decompensated hypothyroidism with inappropriately low FT4 and FT3; E: Disruption of the TSH-T3 feedforward control by monotherapy with L-T4; F and G: Central hypothyroidism with low TSH, FT4 and FT3 concentrations; H: Hypodeiodination in type 1 allostasis (TACITUS/NTIS); I and J: High FT3 in RTH beta and MCT8 deficiency. The grey bar below each panel shows the suggested therapy

10.3 Alternative Biomarkers for Thyroid Hormone Actions

Traditional perspectives regard the TSH concentration as an ideal biomarker of thyroid function since its secretion is very sensitive to changes in FT4 concentration. However, important biological reasons render this approach questionable (see Sect. 10.1.1). Apart from rare diseases (e.g. resistance to thyroid hormone, TSH-secreting adenomas and central hypothyroidism), the TSH concentration may also be misleading in more common conditions, including acute stress, type 1 and type 2 allostatic load and therapy with amiodarone and psychoactive drugs. Additionally, TSH secretion is strongly influenced by circadian and ultradian variations. Unsurprisingly, it was recently demonstrated that free thyroid hormones correlate better with clinical outcomes than the TSH concentration [9]. However, a simple switch to determining thyroid hormone concentrations will not suffice since they may carry some uncertainty as well. This applies especially to conditions of altered plasma protein binding and to patients receiving treatment with levothyroxine or liothyronine, where the hormone concentrations depend on the relative timing of medication intake and lab investigations [29]. *Biomarkers* for thyroid hormone action in tissues may therefore be of additional and complementary interest (Fig. 10.7).

Among those, certain biomarkers that integrate the effect of thyroid hormones over time have turned out to be useful (Table 10.2) [57–59]. Additionally, some *alternative markers* may provide insights into the pathophysiological origins of the metabolic phenotype of thyroid function, thereby providing valuable tools for differential diagnosis and precision therapy [60, 61] (Fig. 10.7, Table 10.2).

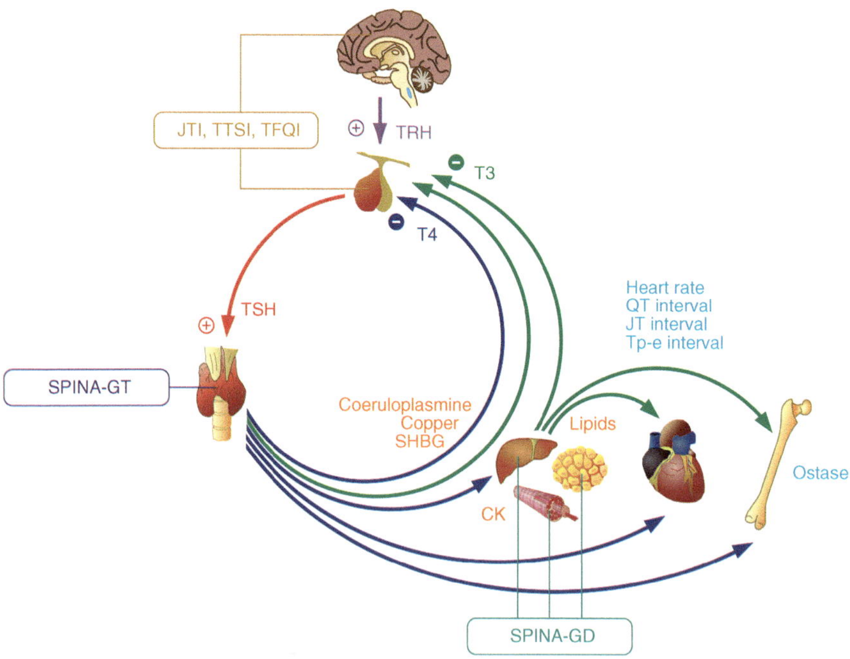

Fig. 10.7 Overview of biomarkers for TR-alpha (cyan) and TR-beta (orange) signalling and of functional biomarkers (rounded boxes)

Table 10.2 Biomarkers for thyroid hormone action in tissues

Positive biomarkers	Negative biomarkers
TR-alpha signalling	
Bone-specific alkaline phosphatase (ostase)	QT interval
Heart rate	JT interval
	Tp-e interval
TR-beta signalling	
3-methylhistidine	Lipids: Total cholesterol, low-density lipoprotein (LDL), high-density lipoprotein (HDL), lipoprotein (a) (Lp(a)), triglycerides
Ceruloplasmin	Creatine kinase (CK)
Copper	
Sex-hormone-binding globulin (SHBG)	

Positive biomarkers increase and negative biomarkers decrease with thyroid hormone signalling

10.3.1 Biochemical Biomarkers

Useful measurable parameters include *indicators for signalling* at TR-alpha and TR-beta receptors. The former group comprises mainly proteins that are produced by the liver under the influence of thyroid hormones, e. g. sex-hormone-binding globulin (SHBG) and ceruloplasmin. Larger concentrations of these proteins reflect the stimulation of protein synthesis by thyroid hormone action. Likewise, concentrations of copper and 3-methylhistidine are positive biomarkers of thyroid function [62, 63]. The concentrations of creatine kinase (CK) and lipids are increased in hypothyroidism and may serve as negative biomarkers of thyroid hormone signalling. This applies especially to concentrations of total cholesterol, low-density lipoprotein (LDL) and triglycerides [64, 65]. High-density lipoprotein (HDL) and lipoprotein (a) Lp(a) concentrations may serve as negative biomarkers as well [66]. Treatment with thyroid hormones may effectively reverse the abnormalities of the lipidomic signature in both subclinical and overt hypothyroidism [67]. The bone-specific alkaline phosphatase (ostase) reflects thyroid hormone signalling in the skeleton. Its serum concentration serves as a biomarker for TR-alpha action and may be used as an additional criterion for dosage titration of thyroid hormone replacement therapy and the monitoring of anti-thyroid treatment in thyrotoxicosis [68].

More recently, *metabolic profiles* and metabolomics have emerged that are able to describe the metabolic state of a hypothyroid or hyperthyroid patient in relation to their thyroid state and treatment response [69, 70].

10.3.2 Electrophysiological Parameters

The heart is among the most important target organs of thyroid hormone signalling. It is therefore not surprising that major adverse cardiovascular events (MACEs) could be related to both hypothyroid and thyrotoxic conditions [50]. Multiple studies observed several intervals in the *electrocardiogram* to reflect the supply of thyroid hormones. The QT, JT and Tp-e intervals, being markers of repolarisation, were positively associated with TSH concentrations and negatively with concentrations of FT4 and FT3 [71–74]. Conversely, the heart rate positively correlates with peripheral thyroid hormone concentrations and negatively with TSH concentration [75].

10.3.3 Neuromonitoring

A traditional symptom of hypothyroidism is a noticeable change in the *Achilles tendon reflex*, particularly a retarded relaxation phase. Accordingly, computer-assisted devices (e.g. patented Thyroflex, Nitek, Scottsdale, AZ, USA) have been developed, aiming to improve the accuracy when assessing the relevant response times after triggering Achilles tendon or brachial reflexes and thereby facilitate a separation of thyroid functional states. Such instruments are not meant to substitute for thyroid function testing but may aid clinical reflexometry and complement the biochemical assessment of a patient.

10.3.4 Calculated Functional Biomarkers

Calculated functional parameters are derived from mathematical models of the homeostatic system [76]. They have been derived to provide mechanistic insights into the pathogenesis of diseases, which help in distinguishing scenarios of superficially similar hormonal phenotypes but different pathophysiological endotypes [33]. Additionally, they provide predictive information for preventive purposes. Functional biomarkers based on calculated properties have been developed for every stage of the feedback loop including the central processing in the hypothalamic–pituitary unit, the thyroid, deiodination and plasma protein binding (Fig. 10.7).

The *thyrotroph thyroid hormone sensitivity index* (*TTSI*) has originally been developed to facilitate screening for classical resistance to thyroid hormone (RTH Beta) [76, 77]. It is also referred to as thyrotroph thyroxine resistance index (TT4RI). This parameter can as well be used as a surrogate marker for the working point of the homeostatic system, e.g. in sepsis and other conditions of severe non-thyroidal illness. It is calculated as

$$\mathrm{TTSI} = \frac{100[\mathrm{TSH}][\mathrm{FT4}]}{l_u}$$

from concentrations of TSH, FT4 and the upper limit of the assay-specific reference interval for the FT4 concentration (l_u). The reference range for the TTSI is between 100 and 150.

A simpler variant omits l_u and calculates TTSI as

$$\mathrm{TTSI} = 100[\mathrm{TSH}][\mathrm{FT4}].$$

We note the results are highly dependent on the respective units of measurement and some properties of the used assays.

The TTSI is elevated in resistance to thyroid hormone and metabolic syndrome, and reduced in situations of inflammation and sepsis. It is sensitive to exposure to endocrine disruptors and may be used for monitoring substitutive therapy with TRIAC in RTHB.

Jostel's TSH index, also referred to as *thyroid function index*, abbreviated TSHI, JTI or TFI, is another marker of the central function of the feedback loop that was primarily developed for the diagnosis of secondary hypothyroidism [76, 78]. It can be calculated as

$$\mathrm{TSHI} = \ln([\mathrm{TSH}]) + \beta[\mathrm{FT4}],$$

where the correction coefficient was determined from population data fitted to a logarithmic function. A z-transformed standardised variant has been described as well. It is obtained with

$$s\mathrm{TSHI} = \frac{\mathrm{TSHI} - 2.7}{0.676}$$

from the mean (2.7) and standard deviation (0.676) of a reference population in the United Kingdom. Reference ranges have been defined to be between 1.3 and 4.1 for the TSHI and, by definition, between −2 and +2 for sTSHI.

This parameter is reduced in thyrotropic insufficiency, but also in situations of a reduced central set point, e.g. in type 1 allostatic load (TACITUS syndrome) and under therapy with certain drugs, e.g. metformin. It is increased in type 2 allostatic load and predicts in this constellation major adverse cardiovascular endpoints (MACEs).

Although both TTSI and TSHI are intended to indicate the thyrotropic function of the hypothalamic–pituitary unit, they deliver slightly different results. This undesired property results from the fact that they have been derived from different models of the negative feedback action.

In order to circumvent this source of distortion, the *thyroid feedback quantile-based index* (*TFQI*) was developed with the aim to provide a more robust and distribution-independent marker of the thyrotropic function [79]. It is obtained with

$$\mathrm{TFQI} = F_{\mathrm{FT4}}([\mathrm{FT4}]) + F_{\mathrm{TSH}}([\mathrm{TSH}]) - 1$$

from the relative positions of the FT4 and TSH concentrations in the respective cumulative distribution functions (F). It has a reference range between −0.74 and +0.74. The TFQI is elevated in psychosocial stress and is positively associated with obesity, metabolic syndrome, type 2 diabetes, diabetes-related complications and all-cause mortality.

The *thyroid's secretory capacity* (also referred to as maximum thyroid hormone output and abbreviated SPINA-GT) is an estimate for the maximum amount of thyroxine that the thyroid gland can produce per second under stimulated conditions. It is derived from a mathematical model of the feedback loop with a "structure parameter inference approach" and delivers a marker for the gain of the thyroid gland (G_T), hence the abbreviation SPINA-GT. It is calculated as

$$\text{SPINA-GT} = \frac{\beta_T \left(D_T + [\text{TSH}]\right)\left(1 + K_{41}[\text{TBG}] + K_{42}[\text{TTR}]\right)[\text{FT4}]}{\alpha_T [\text{TSH}]}$$

from concentrations of TSH and FT4 and some constant parameters for hormone kinetics and dynamics [76]. Its reference range is 1.41–8.67 pmol/s. It is elevated in primary thyrotoxicosis and reduced in primary hypothyroidism, and it correlates with thyroid volume and colour Doppler ultrasound pattern. Its retest reliability is higher than that of TSH, FT4 and FT3 measurements. SPINA-GT has higher sensitivity and specificity for the diagnosis of primary thyrotoxicosis than TSH or thyroid hormones, predicts MACE and overall survival in euthyroid subjects with heart diseases and is critically modified by endocrine disruptors.

The ratio of SPINA-GT and thyroid volume defined by

$$\text{SPINA-GT}_\text{S} = \frac{\text{SPINA} - \text{GT}}{V_T}$$

has been termed *specific thyroid capacity*. It is reduced in obesity and autoimmune thyroiditis [59].

The capacity of step-up deiodination can be estimated by the *sum activity of peripheral deiodinases* (*SPINA-GD*). It represents the maximum amount of T3 that can be produced per second under conditions of substrate saturation. It is calculated as

$$\text{SPINA-GD} = \frac{\beta_{31}\left(K_{M1} + [\text{FT4}]\right)\left(1 + K_{30}[\text{TBG}]\right)[\text{FT3}]}{\alpha_{31}[\text{FT4}]}$$

from concentrations of FT4, FT3 and certain constant parameters. Its reference range is for most assays 20–40 nmol/s. SPINA-GD correlates with isotope-determined conversion from T4 to T3 in slow tissue pools [76]. It is reduced in subacute thyroiditis, exogenous thyrotoxicosis, non-thyroidal illness syndrome (TACITUS) and persons positive for autoantibodies to selenoprotein P. Conversely, it rises after substitution therapy with selenium, a key trace element for the formation of deiodinases, has been started, and it is elevated in conditions of type 2 allostatic load including obesity and metabolic syndrome. SPINA-GD has high specificity for the diagnosis of subacute thyroiditis and, in hypothyroidism, predicts substitution dosage of replacement therapy with levothyroxine [80, 81]. Reduced SPINA-GD is a significant predictor of fatality in trauma and cardiovascular disease [74, 82]. SPINA-GD is quite sensitive to characteristics of the assays used for the determination of FT3. Therefore, a z-transformed standardised version has been developed (SPINA-sGD), to make the results of different assays better comparable.

Of note, all biomarkers are more or less strongly influenced by additional factors beyond thyroid homeostasis, including inflammation, comorbidity, environmental and genetic effects. It is therefore recommended to combine a full profile of thyroid homeostatic evaluation (TSH, FT4, FT3) with several biomarkers to overcome potential biases affecting single parameters.

References

1. Zulewski H, Müller B, Exer P, Miserez AR, Staub JJ. Estimation of tissue hypothyroidism by a new clinical score: evaluation of patients with various grades of hypothyroidism and controls. J Clin Endocrinol Metab. 1997;82:771–6. https://doi.org/10.1210/jcem.82.3.3810.
2. Carlé A, Pedersen IB, Knudsen N, Perrild H, Ovesen L, Andersen S, Laurberg P. Hypothyroid symptoms fail to predict thyroid insufficiency in old people: a population-based case-control study. Am J Med. 2016;129:1082–92. https://doi.org/10.1016/j.amjmed.2016.06.013.
3. Boelaert K, Newby PR, Simmonds MJ, Holder RL, Carr-Smith JD, Heward JM, Manji N, Allahabadia A, Armitage M, Chatterjee KV, Lazarus JH, Pearce SH, Vaidya B, Gough SC, Franklyn JA. Prevalence and relative risk of other autoimmune diseases in subjects with autoimmune thyroid disease. Am J Med. 2010;123(183):e1–9. https://doi.org/10.1016/j.amjmed.2009.06.030.
4. Lakhani OJ, Tripathi S, Indu KC, Desai M. Levothyroxine replacement before glucocorticoid replacement leading to adrenal crisis in a case of autoimmune polyendocrine syndrome type I (Schmidt syndrome). Thyroid Res Pract. 2015;12:116. https://doi.org/10.4103/0973-0354.157932.
5. Karaca Z, Laway BA, Dokmetas HS, Atmaca H, Kelestimur F. Sheehan syndrome. Nat Rev Dis Primers. 2016;2:16092. https://doi.org/10.1038/nrdp.2016.92.
6. Jonklaas J, Bianco AC, Bauer AJ, Burman KD, Cappola AR, Celi FS, Cooper DS, Kim BW, Peeters RP, Rosenthal MS, Sawka AM. Guidelines for the treatment of hypothyroidism: prepared by the American Thyroid Association task force on thyroid hormone replacement. Thyroid. 2014;24:1670–751. https://doi.org/10.1089/thy.2014.0028.
7. Hoermann R, Midgley JEM, Larisch R, Dietrich JW. Advances in applied homeostatic modelling of the relationship between thyrotropin and free thyroxine. PLoS One. 2017;12:e0187232. https://doi.org/10.1371/journal.pone.0187232.
8. Midgley JEM, Toft AD, Larisch R, Dietrich JW, Hoermann R. Time for a reassessment of the treatment of hypothyroidism. BMC Endocr Disord. 2019;19:37. https://doi.org/10.1186/s12902-019-0365-4.
9. Fitzgerald SP, Bean NG, Falhammar H, Tuke J. Clinical parameters are more likely to be associated with thyroid hormone levels than with thyrotropin levels: a systematic review and meta-analysis. Thyroid. 2020;30:1695–709. https://doi.org/10.1089/thy.2019.0535.
10. Dietrich JW, Landgrafe G, Fotiadou EH. TSH and thyrotropic agonists: key actors in thyroid homeostasis. J Thyroid Res. 2012;2012:351864. https://doi.org/10.1155/2012/351864.
11. Hoermann R, Midgley JEM, Larisch R, Dietrich JW. Relational stability in the expression of normality, variation, and control of thyroid function. Front Endocrinol (Lausanne). 2016;7:142. https://doi.org/10.3389/fendo.2016.00142.

12. Fitzgerald SP, Bean NG, Falhammar H, Hoermann R. Physiological linkage of thyroid and pituitary sensitivities. Endocrine. 2023;79:143–51. https://doi.org/10.1007/s12020-022-03184-8.
13. Surks MI, Goswami G, Daniels GH. The thyrotropin reference range should remain unchanged. J Clin Endocrinol Metab. 2005;90:5489–96. https://doi.org/10.1210/jc.2005-0170.
14. Wartofsky L, Dickey RA. The evidence for a narrower thyrotropin reference range is compelling. J Clin Endocrinol Metab. 2005;90:5483–8. https://doi.org/10.1210/jc.2005-0455.
15. Dickey RA, Wartofsky L, Feld S. Optimal thyrotropin level: normal ranges and reference intervals are not equivalent. Thyroid. 2005;15:1035–9. https://doi.org/10.1089/thy.2005.15.1035.
16. Völzke H, Alte D, Kohlmann T, Lüdemann J, Nauck M, John U, Meng W. Reference intervals of serum thyroid function tests in a previously iodine-deficient area. Thyroid. 2005;15:279–85. https://doi.org/10.1089/thy.2005.15.279.
17. Laurberg P, Andersen S, Carlé A, Karmisholt J, Knudsen N, Pedersen IB. The TSH upper reference limit: where are we at? Nat Rev Endocrinol. 2011;7:232–9. https://doi.org/10.1038/nrendo.2011.13.
18. Jonklaas J, Razvi S. Reference intervals in the diagnosis of thyroid dysfunction: treating patients not numbers. Lancet Diabetes Endocrinol. 2019;7:473–83. https://doi.org/10.1016/S2213-8587(18)30371-1.
19. Walsh JP. Thyroid function across the lifespan: do age-related changes matter. Endocrinol Metab (Seoul). 2022;37:208–19. https://doi.org/10.3803/EnM.2022.1463.
20. Van Uytfanghe K, Ehrenkranz J, Halsall D, Hoff K, Loh TP, Spencer CA, Köhrle J. Thyroid stimulating hormone and thyroid hormones (triiodothyronine and thyroxine): an American Thyroid Association-commissioned review of current clinical and laboratory status. Thyroid. 2023;33:1013–28. https://doi.org/10.1089/thy.2023.0169.
21. Jonklaas J. TSH reference intervals: their importance and complexity. Thyroid. 2024; https://doi.org/10.1089/thy.2024.0380.
22. Andersen S, Pedersen KM, Bruun NH, Laurberg P. Narrow individual variations in serum T4 and T3 in normal subjects: a clue to the understanding of subclinical thyroid disease. J Clin Endocrinol Metab. 2002;87:1068–72. https://doi.org/10.1210/jcem.87.3.8165.
23. Hoermann R, Midgley JEM, Larisch R, Dietrich JW. Individualised requirements for optimum treatment of hypothyroidism: complex needs, limited options. Drugs Context. 2019;8:212597. https://doi.org/10.7573/dic.212597.
24. Hoermann R, Midgley JEM, Larisch R, Dietrich JW. Functional and symptomatic individuality in the response to levothyroxine treatment. Front Endocrinol (Lausanne). 2019;10:664. https://doi.org/10.3389/fendo.2019.00664.
25. Hoermann R, Eckl WA, Hoermann C, Larisch R. Complex relationship between free thyroxine and TSH in the regulation of thyroid function. Eur J Endocrinol. 2010;162:1123–9. https://doi.org/10.1530/EJE-10-0106.
26. Clark PM, Holder RL, Haque SM, Hobbs FD, Roberts LM, Franklyn JA. The relationship between serum TSH and free T4 in older people. J Clin Pathol. 2012;65:463–5. https://doi.org/10.1136/jclinpath-2011-200433.
27. Hadlow NC, Rothacker KM, Wardrop R, Brown SJ, Lim EM, Walsh JP. The relationship between TSH and free t4 in a large population is complex and nonlinear and differs by age and sex. J Clin Endocrinol Metab. 2013;98:2936–43. https://doi.org/10.1210/jc.2012-4223.
28. Midgley JEM, Hoermann R, Larisch R, Dietrich JW. Physiological states and functional relation between thyrotropin and free thyroxine in thyroid health and disease: in vivo and in silico data suggest a hierarchical model. J Clin Pathol. 2013;66:335–42. https://doi.org/10.1136/jclinpath-2012-201213.
29. Hoermann R, Midgley JEM, Giacobino A, Eckl WA, Wahl HG, Dietrich JW, Larisch R. Homeostatic equilibria between free thyroid hormones and pituitary thyrotropin are modulated by various influences including age, body mass index and treatment. Clin Endocrinol. 2014;81:907–15. https://doi.org/10.1111/cen.12527.

30. Korem Kohanim Y, Milo T, Raz M, Karin O, Bar A, Mayo A, Mendelson Cohen N, Toledano Y, Alon U. Dynamics of thyroid diseases and thyroid-axis gland masses. Mol Syst Biol. 2022;18:e10919. https://doi.org/10.15252/msb.202210919.
31. Rücker G, Schumacher M. Simpson's paradox visualized: the example of the rosiglitazone meta-analysis. BMC Med Res Methodol. 2008;8:34. https://doi.org/10.1186/1471-2288-8-34.
32. Hamaker EL. Why researchers should think "within-person": a paradigmatic rationale. In: Mehl MR, Conner TS, editors. Handbook of research methods for studying daily life. New York: Guilford Press; 2012. p. 43–61.
33. Hoermann R, Midgley JEM, Larisch R, Dietrich JW. Lessons from randomised clinical trials for triiodothyronine treatment of hypothyroidism: have they achieved their objectives. J Thyroid Res. 2018;2018:3239197. https://doi.org/10.1155/2018/3239197.
34. Fisher AJ, Medaglia JD, Jeronimus BF. Lack of group-to-individual generalizability is a threat to human subjects research. Proc Natl Acad Sci USA. 2018;115:E6106–15. https://doi.org/10.1073/pnas.1711978115.
35. Spencer CA, Lopresti JS, Patel A, Guttler RB, Eigen A, Shen D, Gray D, Nicoloff JT. Applications of a new chemiluminometric thyrotropin assay to subnormal measurement. J Clin Endocrinol Metab. 1990;70:453–60. https://doi.org/10.1210/jcem-70-2-453.
36. Baloch Z, Carayon P, Conte-Devolx B, Demers LM, Feldt-Rasmussen U, Henry JF, Livosli VA, Niccoli-Sire P, John R, Ruf J, Smyth PP, Spencer CA, Stockigt JR, Guidelines Committee NAOCB. Laboratory medicine practice guidelines. Laboratory support for the diagnosis and monitoring of thyroid disease. Thyroid. 2004;13:3–126. https://doi.org/10.1089/105072503321086962.
37. Benhadi N, Fliers E, Visser TJ, Reitsma JB, Wiersinga WM. Pilot study on the assessment of the setpoint of the hypothalamus-pituitary-thyroid axis in healthy volunteers. Eur J Endocrinol. 2010;162:323–9. https://doi.org/10.1530/EJE-09-0655.
38. Leow MKS. The TSH-free thyroxine relationship: logarithmic—linear or error function? Eur J Endocrinol. 2010;163:839–40. https://doi.org/10.1530/EJE-10-0675.
39. Van Deventer HE, Mendu DR, Remaley AT, Soldin SJ. Inverse log-linear relationship between thyroid-stimulating hormone and free thyroxine measured by direct analog immunoassay and tandem mass spectrometry. Clin Chem. 2011;57:122–7. https://doi.org/10.1373/clinchem.2010.154088.
40. Raz M, Milo T, Glass DS, Mayo A, Alon U. Endocrine gland size is proportional to its target tissue size. iScience. 2024;27(9):110625. https://doi.org/10.1016/j.isci.2024.110625.
41. Hoermann R, Midgley JEM, Larisch R, Dietrich JW. Treatment options for subclinical hypothyroidism. Eur J Endocrinol. 2021;185:L5–6. https://doi.org/10.1530/EJE-20-1405.
42. Peeters RP, Brito JP. Subclinical hypothyroidism: to treat or not to treat. Eur J Endocrinol. 2020;183:D15–24. https://doi.org/10.1530/EJE-20-0621.
43. Peterson SJ, Cappola AR, Castro MR, Dayan CM, Farwell AP, Hennessey JV, Kopp PA, Ross DS, Samuels MH, Sawka AM, Taylor PN, Jonklaas J, Bianco AC. An online survey of hypothyroid patients demonstrates prominent dissatisfaction. Thyroid. 2018;28:707–21. https://doi.org/10.1089/thy.2017.0681.
44. Molewijk E, Fliers E, Dreijerink K, Van Dooren A, Heerdink R. Quality of life, daily functioning, and symptoms in hypothyroid patients on thyroid replacement therapy: a Dutch survey. J Clin Transl Endocrinol. 2024;35:100330. https://doi.org/10.1016/j.jcte.2024.100330.
45. Hoermann R, Pekker M, Midgley JEM, Larisch R, Dietrich JW. Principles of endocrine regulation: reconciling tensions between robustness in performance and adaptation to change. Front Endocrinol (Lausanne). 2022;13:825107. https://doi.org/10.3389/fendo.2022.825107.
46. Hoermann R, Pekker MJ, Midgley JEM, Dietrich JW. The role of supporting and disruptive mechanisms of FT3 homeostasis in regulating the hypothalamic-pituitary-thyroid axis. Ther Adv Endocrinol Metab. 2023;14:20420188231158163. https://doi.org/10.1177/20420188231158163.
47. Biondi B, Cooper DS. The clinical significance of subclinical thyroid dysfunction. Endocr Rev. 2008;29:76–131. https://doi.org/10.1210/er.2006-0043.

48. Cooper DS, Biondi B. Subclinical thyroid disease. Lancet. 2012;379:1142–54. https://doi.org/10.1016/S0140-6736(11)60276-6.
49. Dietrich JW, Hoermann R, Midgley JEM, Bergen F, Müller P. The two faces of Janus: why thyrotropin as a cardiovascular risk factor may be an ambiguous target. Front Endocrinol (Lausanne). 2020;11:829. https://doi.org/10.3389/fendo.2020.542710.
50. Müller P, Leow MK, Dietrich JW. Minor perturbations of thyroid homeostasis and major cardiovascular endpoints-physiological mechanisms and clinical evidence. Front Cardiovasc Med. 2022;9:942971. https://doi.org/10.3389/fcvm.2022.942971.
51. Peeters RP, Van Toor H, Klootwijk W, De Rijke YB, Kuiper GG, Uitterlinden AG, Visser TJ. Polymorphisms in thyroid hormone pathway genes are associated with plasma TSH and iodothyronine levels in healthy subjects. J Clin Endocrinol Metab. 2003;88:2880–8. https://doi.org/10.1210/jc.2002-021592.
52. Dayan CM, Panicker V. Novel insights into thyroid hormones from the study of common genetic variation. Nat Rev Endocrinol. 2009;5:211–8. https://doi.org/10.1038/nrendo.2009.19.
53. Medici M, Visser WE, Visser TJ, Peeters RP. Genetic determination of the hypothalamic-pituitary-thyroid axis: where do we stand? Endocr Rev. 2015;36:214–44. https://doi.org/10.1210/er.2014-1081.
54. Carlé A, Faber J, Steffensen R, Laurberg P, Nygaard B. Hypothyroid patients encoding combined MCT10 and dio2 gene polymorphisms may prefer L-T3 + L-T4 combination treatment—data using a blind, randomized, clinical study. Eur Thyroid J. 2017;6:143–51. https://doi.org/10.1159/000469709.
55. Bianco AC, Kim BS. Pathophysiological relevance of deiodinase polymorphism. Curr Opin Endocrinol Diabetes Obes. 2018;25:341–6. https://doi.org/10.1097/MED.0000000000000428.
56. Sterenborg RBTM, Steinbrenner I, Li Y, Bujnis MN, Naito T, Marouli E, Galesloot TE, Babajide O, Andreasen L, Astrup A, Åsvold BO, Bandinelli S, Beekman M, Beilby JP, Bork-Jensen J, Boutin T, Brody JA, Brown SJ, Brumpton B, Campbell PJ, Cappola AR, Ceresini G, Chaker L, Chasman DI, Concas MP, Coutinho De Almeida R, Cross SM, Cucca F, Deary IJ, Kjaergaard AD, Echouffo Tcheugui JB, Ellervik C, Eriksson JG, Ferrucci L, Freudenberg J, Ghs D, Regeneron GC, Fuchsberger C, Gieger C, Giulianini F, Gögele M, Graham SE, Grarup N, Gunjača I, Hansen T, Harding BN, Harris SE, Haunsø S, Hayward C, Hui J, Ittermann T, Jukema JW, Kajantie E, Kanters JK, Kårhus LL, Kiemeney LALM, Kloppenburg M, Kühnel B, Lahti J, Langenberg C, Lapauw B, Leese G, Li S, Liewald DCM, Linneberg A, Lominchar JVT, Luan J, Martin NG, Matana A, Meima ME, Meitinger T, Meulenbelt I, Mitchell BD, Møllehave LT, Mora S, Naitza S, Nauck M, Netea-Maier RT, Noordam R, Nursyifa C, Okada Y, Onano S, Papadopoulou A, Palmer CNA, Pattaro C, Pedersen O, Peters A, Pietzner M, Polašek O, Pramstaller PP, Psaty BM, Punda A, Ray D, Redmond P, Richards JB, Ridker PM, Russ TC, Ryan KA, Olesen MS, Schultheiss UT, Selvin E, Siddiqui MK, Sidore C, Slagboom PE, Sørensen TIA, Soto-Pedre E, Spector TD, Spedicati B, Srinivasan S, Starr JM, Stott DJ, Tanaka T, Torlak V, Trompet S, Tuhkanen J, Uitterlinden AG, Van Den Akker EB, Van Den Eynde T, Van Der Klauw MM, Van Heemst D, Verroken C, Visser WE, Vojinovic D, Völzke H, Waldenberger M, Walsh JP, Wareham NJ, Weiss S, Willer CJ, Wilson SG, Wolffenbuttel BHR, Wouters HJCM, Wright MJ, Yang Q, Zemunik T, Zhou W, Zhu G, Zöllner S, Smit JWA, Peeters RP, Köttgen A, Teumer A, Medici M. Multi-trait analysis characterizes the genetics of thyroid function and identifies causal associations with clinical implications. Nat Commun. 2024;15:888. https://doi.org/10.1038/s41467-024-44701-9.
57. Beck-Peccoz P, Lania A, Beckers A, Chatterjee K, Wemeau JL. 2013 European Thyroid Association guidelines for the diagnosis and treatment of thyrotropin-secreting pituitary tumors. Eur Thyroid J. 2013;2:76–82. https://doi.org/10.1159/000351007.
58. Ito M, Miyauchi A, Hisakado M, Yoshioka W, Ide A, Kudo T, Nishihara E, Kihara M, Ito Y, Kobayashi K, Miya A, Fukata S, Nishikawa M, Nakamura H, Amino N. Biochemical markers reflecting thyroid function in athyreotic patients on levothyroxine monotherapy. Thyroid. 2017;27:484–90. https://doi.org/10.1089/thy.2016.0426.

59. Hoermann R, Midgley JEM, Larisch R, Dietrich JW. Relational stability of thyroid hormones in euthyroid subjects and patients with autoimmune thyroid disease. Eur Thyroid J. 2016;5:171–9. https://doi.org/10.1159/000447967.
60. Fitzgerald SP, Falhammar H. Redefinition of successful treatment of patients with hypothyroidism. Is TSH the best biomarker of euthyroidism. Front Endocrinol (Lausanne). 2022;13:920854. https://doi.org/10.3389/fendo.2022.920854.
61. Jansen HI, Bruinstroop E, Heijboer AC, Boelen A. Biomarkers indicating tissue thyroid hormone status: ready to be implemented yet? J Endocrinol. 2022;253:R21–45. https://doi.org/10.1530/JOE-21-0364.
62. Rodier M, Richard JL, Bringer J, Cavalié G, Bellet H, Mirouze J. Thyroid status and muscle protein breakdown as assessed by urinary 3-methylhistidine excretion: study in thyrotoxic patients before and after treatment. Metabolism. 1984;33:97–100. https://doi.org/10.1016/0026-0495(84)90169-0.
63. Mittag J, Behrends T, Nordström K, Anselmo J, Vennström B, Schomburg L. Serum copper as a novel biomarker for resistance to thyroid hormone. Biochem J. 2012;443:103–9. https://doi.org/10.1042/BJ20111817.
64. Nikkilä EA, Kekki M. Plasma triglyceride metabolism in thyroid disease. J Clin Invest. 1972;51:2103–14. https://doi.org/10.1172/JCI107017.
65. Lithell H, Boberg J, Hellsing K, Ljunghall S, Lundqvist G, Vessby B, Wide L. Serum lipoprotein and apolipoprotein concentrations and tissue lipoprotein-lipase activity in overt and subclinical hypothyroidism: the effect of substitution therapy. Eur J Clin Investig. 1981;11:3–10. https://doi.org/10.1111/j.1365-2362.1981.tb01758.x.
66. Rizos CV, Elisaf MS, Liberopoulos EN. Effects of thyroid dysfunction on lipid profile. Open Cardiovasc Med J. 2011;5:76–84. https://doi.org/10.2174/1874192401105010076.
67. Jonklaas J. Hypothyroidism, lipids, and lipidomics. Endocrine. 2023; https://doi.org/10.1007/s12020-023-03420-9.
68. Boruah P, Baruah AJ, Hajong R, Nath CK, Barman B, Chutia H, Sarma K. A study to assess the validity of estimation of serum ostase level in hyperthyroid and hypothyroid cases. J Clin Diagn Res. 2016;10:BC08–11. https://doi.org/10.7860/JCDR/2016/19750.8441.
69. Piras C, Pibiri M, Leoni VP, Balsamo A, Tronci L, Arisci N, Mariotti S, Atzori L. Analysis of metabolomics profile in hypothyroid patients before and after thyroid hormone replacement. J Endocrinol Investig. 2021;44:1309–19. https://doi.org/10.1007/s40618-020-01434-y.
70. Jaber MA, Benabdelkamel H, Dahabiyeh LA, Masood A, Almalki RH, Musambil M, Alfadda AA, Abdel Rahman AM. The metabolomics approach revealed a distinctive metabolomics pattern associated with hyperthyroidism treatment. Front Endocrinol (Lausanne). 2022;13:1050201. https://doi.org/10.3389/fendo.2022.1050201.
71. Galetta F, Franzoni F, Fallahi P, Tocchini L, Braccini L, Santoro G, Antonelli A. Changes in heart rate variability and qt dispersion in patients with overt hypothyroidism. Eur J Endocrinol. 2008;158:85–90. https://doi.org/10.1530/EJE-07-0357.
72. Gürdal A, Eroğlu H, Helvaci F, Sümerkan MÇ, Kasali K, Çetin Ş, Aksan G, Kiliçkesmez K. Evaluation of tp-e interval, tp-e/qt ratio and tp-e/qtc ratio in patients with subclinical hypothyroidism. Ther Adv Endocrinol Metab. 2017;8:25–32. https://doi.org/10.1177/2042018816684423.
73. Madhukar R, Jagadeesh AT, Moey MYY, Vaglio M, Badilini F, Leban M, Hartemann A, Dureau P, Funck-Brentano C, Bourron O, Salem JE. Association of thyroid-stimulating hormone with corrected qt interval variation: a prospective cohort study among patients with type 2 diabetes. Arch Cardiovasc Dis. 2021;114:656–66. https://doi.org/10.1016/j.acvd.2021.06.008.
74. Aweimer A, Dietrich JW, Santoro F, Fàbregas MC, Mügge A, Núñez-Gil IJ, Vazirani R, Vedia O, Pätz T, Ragnatela I. Takotsubo syndrome outcomes predicted by thyroid hormone signature: insights from cluster analysis of a multicentre registry. EBioMedicine. 2024;102:105063. https://doi.org/10.1016/j.ebiom.2024.105063.

75. Aweimer A, Schiedat F, Schöne D, Landgrafe-Mende G, Bogossian H, Mügge A, Patsalis PC, Gotzmann M, Akin I, El-Battrawy I, Dietrich JW. Abnormal cardiac repolarization in thyroid diseases: results of an observational study. Front Cardiovasc Med. 2021;8:738517. https://doi.org/10.3389/fcvm.2021.738517.
76. Dietrich JW, Landgrafe-Mende G, Wiora E, Chatzitomaris A, Klein HH, Midgley JEM, Hoermann R. Calculated parameters of thyroid homeostasis: emerging tools for differential diagnosis and clinical research. Front Endocrinol (Lausanne). 2016;7:57. https://doi.org/10.3389/fendo.2016.00057.
77. Yagi H, Pohlenz J, Hayashi Y, Sakurai A, Refetoff S. Resistance to thyroid hormone caused by two mutant thyroid hormone receptors beta, r243q and r243w, with marked impairment of function that cannot be explained by altered in vitro 3,5,3'-triiodothyronine binding affinity. J Clin Endocrinol Metab. 1997;82:1608–14. https://doi.org/10.1210/jcem.82.5.3945.
78. Jostel A, Ryder WDJ, Shalet SM. The use of thyroid function tests in the diagnosis of hypopituitarism: definition and evaluation of the TSH index. Clin Endocrinol. 2009;71:529–34. https://doi.org/10.1111/j.1365-2265.2009.03534.x.
79. Laclaustra M, Moreno-Franco B, Lou-Bonafonte JM, Mateo-Gallego R, Casasnovas JA, Guallar-Castillon P, Cenarro A, Civeira F. Impaired sensitivity to thyroid hormones is associated with diabetes and metabolic syndrome. Diabetes Care. 2019;42:303–10. https://doi.org/10.2337/dc18-1410.
80. Midgley JEM, Larisch R, Dietrich JW, Hoermann R. Variation in the biochemical response to L-thyroxine therapy and relationship with peripheral thyroid hormone conversion efficiency. Endocr Connect. 2015;4:196–205. https://doi.org/10.1530/EC-15-0056.
81. Le Moli R, Malandrino P, Russo M, Tumino D, Piticchio T, Naselli A, Rapicavoli V, Belfiore A, Frasca F. Levothyroxine therapy, calculated deiodinases activity and basal metabolic rate in obese or nonobese patients after total thyroidectomy for differentiated thyroid cancer, results of a retrospective observational study. Endocrinol Diabetes Metab. 2023;6(2):e406. https://doi.org/10.1002/edm2.406.
82. Dietrich JW, Ackermann A, Kasippillai A, Kanthasamy Y, Tharmalingam T, Urban A, Vasileva S, Schildhauer TA, Klein HH, Stachon A, Hering S. Adaptive veränderungen des schilddrüsenstoffwechsels als risikoindikatoren bei traumata. Trauma Berufskrankh. 2019:1–8. https://doi.org/10.1007/s10039-019-00438-z.

Chapter 11
Treatment of Hypothyroidism

Rudolf Hoermann and Johannes W. Dietrich

Treatment of hypothyroidism relies on the principle of *hormone substitution* through external administration of thyroid hormones when the patient's own thyroid gland can no longer produce them in sufficient quantities [1, 2]. This permits the normal functioning of the many thyroid hormone-dependent reactions and metabolic actions. Physiologically, the human thyroid gland produces mainly *two thyroid hormones*, a large amount of T4 and a much lesser amount of T3 (Chap. 3). Both hormones are *stored* in the follicular structure of the gland to be readily available and released on-demand in a controlled way (Chap. 5). The storage capability of the thyroid gland is different from other endocrine glands, such as the adrenals or testes, which cannot rely on stored hormone depots. This unique feature of the thyroid gland makes the supply of the body with thyroid hormones less dependent on nutritional variations in iodine supply, provisional and through its regulation anticipatory of demand. In the thyroid system, the two main hormones, T4 and T3, have different properties and differentiated roles. While T4 is exclusively synthesised by the

R. Hoermann (✉)
Yandina, QLD, Australia

Department of General Internal Medicine, Gastroenterology and Endocrinology, [Retired] Klinikum Lüdenscheid, Lüdenscheid, Germany
e-mail: rudolf.hoermann@gmail.com

J. W. Dietrich
Diabetes, Endocrinology and Metabolism Section, Department of Medicine, St. Josef-Hospital, Ruhr University Hospitals, Bochum, Germany

Centre for Diabetes Technology (ZDT), Catholic Hospitals Bochum, Bochum, Germany

Centre for Rare Endocrine Diseases (ZSEK), Ruhr Center for Rare Diseases (CeSER), Ruhr University of Bochum and Witten/Herdecke University, Bochum, Germany

Centre for Thyroid Medicine (ZSM), Ruhr University of Bochum, Bochum, Germany
e-mail: johannes.dietrich@ruhr-uni-bochum.de

R. Hoermann, J. W. Dietrich (eds.), *Hypothyroidism*,
https://doi.org/10.1007/978-981-96-3682-2_11

thyroid, dependent on appropriate and controlled glandular stimulation by the pituitary hormone, thyroid-stimulating hormone (TSH), T3 is only partly synthesised there and generated to a much larger extent locally in many other tissues via enzymatic monodeiodination of T4. Notably, the proportion of intra-thyroidal and extra-thyroidal T3 production is not fixed, as often falsely assumed, but adapts to different conditions [3]. In this regard, an important study has been carried out in rats [4]. With their fully functioning thyroid still in place, the animals were even able to survive under experimental conditions of a deficiency in all three types of deiodinases and the total loss of extra-thyroidal T3 generation by the enzymes [4]. Given the conversion of T4 to T3 and activation of the former to a molecule of enhanced potency, T4 is regarded as a precursor to T3. The intra-thyroidal formation of T3 from its precursor T4 is subject to feed-forward regulation by pituitary TSH, as is thyroidal T3 secretion [5–9]. The *pleiotropic signalling through TSH* provides unexpected system-level functionality to the hypothalamic–pituitary–thyroid axis regulation [9] (see Chap. 5). It supports robustness of the system, allowing for the maintenance of FT3 homeostasis despite changes in the availability of its precursor FT4. While the actions of FT4 and TSH oppose each other in the regulation of the hypothalamic–pituitary–thyroid axis, they combine and join forces to maintain FT3 concentration at a homeostatic level [9]. The clinical relevance has already been discussed when introducing the concept of *relational stability (Chap.* 2) This design of control is not unique to hypothalamic–pituitary–thyroid regulation, but more generally operative in growth control via two hormones (human growth hormone and insulin-like growth factor 1) and cellular circuits with *incomplete feed-forward loops of control* by "paradoxical" components [10].

Our view on the role of the seemingly minor, putatively negligible, thyroidal co-secretion of T3 with T4 has been fundamentally changed by these more recent findings [11]. They suggested a regulatory *role of glandular T3 production* that exceeds its quantitative contribution to the thyroid hormone pool. Accordingly, functional thyroid capacity and adaptive T3 generation are both integral elements in providing balanced system stability and adjusting the sensitivity of hypothalamic–pituitary–thyroid feedback control, as detailed in Chaps. 2 and 5. In athyreotic patients on levothyroxine monotherapy, on the other hand, the loss of stabilising mechanisms in the absence of a functioning thyroid may explain an observed homeostatic instability in the FT3 levels [11]. The behaviour of FT3 levels in athyreotic patients is in sharp contrast to the FT3 stability observed over a wide range of TSH values in subjects with a fully functioning thyroid gland [11] (see Chap. 2).

Historically, *thyroid hormone replacement* was successfully introduced with the application of *animal thyroid extracts* of ovine, bovine or porcine source [12–16]. This was enabled by the unique property of the thyroid as a storage organ, as opposed to other endocrine glands relying on ad-hoc synthesis of hormones. These non-human thyroid extracts contain a relatively larger amount of T3, compared to the human thyroid [17]. While desiccated thyroid hormone extracts remain a popular treatment choice among hypothyroid patients in the United States even today [18], in most parts of the world a shift occurred in the standard treatment strategy towards the use of *synthetic levothyroxine* (*LT4*) *drugs* and *LT4 monotherapy* [15].

This decision, though not based on formal trials, was guided by several *assumptions* and events.

First, a shift in the definition of hypothyroidism focused on the T4-based supply side of the hormone in primary hypothyroidism, while considering the minor contribution and complementary role of glandular T3 secretion to be negligible [19]. This view caused a shift in the diagnosis of hypothyroidism relying primarily on TSH measurement, complemented by FT4, with FT3 evaluation being regarded as redundant. The strategy has been backed by a simplistic view on the hypothalamic–pituitary–thyroid axis control, particularly the classical models of the pituitary-thyroid subsystem or TSH-FT4 regulation, but disregarded the more complex implications of a T3-inclusive system of the regulation (Chaps. 2 and 5).

Second, it relied on the unproven assumption of *T3 autonomy* of peripheral tissues, in that T3 would always be generated as needed by the local processes, provided a sufficient amount of its prohormone T4 is made available. Clinical acceptance rests on an *undue generalisation* of several randomised controlled studies and meta-analyses which failed to demonstrate a superiority of LT4/LT3 combination drugs over LT4 monotherapy [20–23].

Third, the *favourable pharmacological* profile of long-acting levothyroxine drugs and a fear of adverse T3 reactions made administration of the prohormone T4 a presumed safer option.

The role of T3 in the diagnosis and treatment of hypothyroidism has only recently gained *renewed interest* after patients increasingly voiced their concerns and dissatisfaction with the standard treatment. Their sentiment was confirmed by a large *online survey* conducted by the American Thyroid Association [24]. It is shared by many practitioners around the globe. A Dutch survey came to the same conclusion [25]. This study included controls, and a majority of patients (52%) had lower FT3 concentrations. Evidence has accumulated that standard levothyroxine monotherapy may not suit the needs of all patients with hypothyroidism, but leaving a substantial portion of patients with residual symptoms despite achieving the guideline-endorsed target of "normalisation" of their TSH levels [26–29]. An advanced understanding of hypothalamic–pituitary–thyroid regulation predicts and explains these particularities and encourages reconsideration of T3/T4 combination therapy (Chap. 5). Before we address these issues, it may be appropriate to review the treatment goals and established standards of therapy for patients with hypothyroidism.

11.1 Treatment Goals

The *treatment goals* for a hypothyroid patient are dual, aiming at both the relief of hypothyroid clinical symptoms and biochemical normalisation of thyroid function to restore euthyroidism, as best as possible.

Hence, main goals in the treatment of hypothyroidism are

1. Relief form hypothyroid symptoms
2. Restoration of general well-being
3. Achievement of biochemical euthyroidism
4. Avoidance of hyperthyroid symptoms and over-treatment

11.1.1 Whom to Treat

Before treatment can be initiated to a patient, the diagnosis of hypothyroidism must be established and *confirmed* (Chap. 10). This is readily achieved in patients presenting with symptomatic overt hypothyroidism, by means of the patient's history, presenting complaints, clinical examination of signs of hypothyroidism and biochemical thyroid function testing. In a typical patient with primary hypothyroidism, the latter will readily document a low FT4 concentration together with a markedly elevated TSH level. In secondary hypothyroidism, FT4 measurement remains a reliable parameter, whereas TSH provides little diagnostic value. Due to the pituitary failure, TSH concentration can be low, within its reference range or sometimes even moderately elevated. As an indication, TSH is found to be *inappropriate* relative to the low FT4 concentration. Abnormal results of other pituitary hormones may further aid in confirming the diagnosis of the pituitary disease (Fig. 10.6).

However, asymptomatic patients with the biochemical constellation of *subclinical hypothyroidism* are far more prevalent. They present a greater diagnostic and therapeutic challenge. The definition and diagnostic uncertainties of this *laboratory constellation* have been discussed (Chap. 8). *Additional criteria* are required in subclinical hypothyroidism to determine whether the patient may be truly hypothyroid and in need of medical intervention. Any *treatment decision* has to be made individually on a case-by-case basis, taking clinical and biochemical markers of disease into account [30].

The same is true for *rare causes* of hypothyroidism that may not fall into readily recognisable diagnostic categories. In particular, syndromes of insensitivity to thyroid hormone (including MCT8 deficiency) and non-thyroidal illness present serious diagnostic and therapeutic challenges.

11.1.2 How to Treat Hypothyroidism

Since the 1970s the standard mode of treating hypothyroidism has been the replacement of the main thyroid hormone as a levothyroxine *(LT4) drug* [1, 2, 19, 31]. The *LT4 drug* has important properties to support the safety of treatment, i.e. surviving in the circulation for a prolonged time, with a plasma half-life of approx. 7 days, and acting as a precursor to the biologically more active T3 hormone, allowing for the generation of T3 via enzymatic monodeiodination at the level of many tissues. The choice of the *standard treatment is different from the natural situation*, where the human thyroid co-secretes T3 together with T4, albeit in a lesser amount, compared to the much larger production of the latter. Daily production rates have been estimated to amount to approx. 100 μg/day of T4 and 10 μg/day of T3 [32].

Consequently, the rationale for using LT4 monotherapy as the current treatment of choice in hypothyroidism did not remain unchallenged. A number of studies and meta-analyses were conducted in the past, comparing LT4 monotherapy with LT3/LT4 combinations [20–22, 33]. Attempts to prove the *superiority* of either one of the two options failed. This has been used as a strong argument by advocates in favour of LT4 monotherapy. It helped elevate LT4 monotherapy to its current position as the guideline-endorsed standard treatment of hypothyroidism [1, 19]. However, the inadequacies of this process must be considered [22]. Among other *caveats*, there are issues with the universality of the approach and more specifically these studies that have long been dismissed. More recent studies attempted to bring the FT3 to FT4 ratio into the physiological range with TSH-adjusted LT4 treatment but did not find superior efficacy, compared to LT4 monotherapy, in this setting of a randomised double-blind design [34]. These analyses are still lacking statistical rigour, for instance not considering intraclass correlations and Simpson's paradox in the expression of high individuality by thyroid hormones [35].

11.1.3 Treatment Modality

The LT4 drug is typically *taken orally as a single morning dose*, administered once daily 30 min before breakfast [36]. This permits optimum gastrointestinal absorption of the hormone. Alternatively, the drug can be taken with a minor dose increase with some food at breakfast, which is subjectively preferred by some patients. Other patients may opt for evening ingestion or divided dosing (bid). Due to the prolonged half-life of the LT4 drug in the blood stream, differences between these regimes remain marginal and uncritical in most patients [37]. The choice is optional, as long as appropriate and stable treatment targets can be achieved.

11.1.4 Dose Finding

Hormones such as levothyroxine cannot be administered in a fixed standard dose, unlike many other drugs. Rather the appropriate dose is highly individual and is *to be determined for each patient* [1, 19, 30]. It needs to be further *adjusted* if circumstances change. *Dose adequacy* is guided by residual complaints and symptoms of the patient, possible hyperthyroid signs of overdosing of the drug together with the results of biochemical testing.

Blood samples for testing should best be obtained *before* the drug is ingested, but not shortly after the administration of the LT4 dose, as this may lead to a temporary minor increase in FT4 serum concentrations. Because of *diurnal variation* in the circulating concentrations of TSH levels, blood sampling should best be performed in the morning [38].

The average *daily dose* of LT4 required depends on the body weight of the patient, being approx. 1.6 µg/kg body weight/day or 100–150 µg LT4/day. Otherwise healthy patients can start on their full target dose from the beginning of the treatment. Older patients and patients with coronary heart disease are advised to begin more cautiously, increasing the dose after 4 weeks if it is well tolerated.

LT4 dose requirement may moderately decrease in older people. Women during *pregnancy* or when taking oral contraceptives must increase their regular LT4 dose, mostly by approx. 50 µg LT4/day (Chap. 12).

The most severe form of hypothyroidism, *myxedematous coma* is an emergency situation, where high doses of LT4 are required and must be administered intravenously [39].

Patients with *secondary hypothyroidism* require on average slightly lower LT4 doses, compared to patients with primary hypothyroidism, because low-level basal secretion of thyroid hormones by the thyroid is still present and contributing to the hormone pool. TSH measurement is unable to guide dose finding in secondary hypothyroidism, with only FT4 and FT3 concentrations being useful to monitor this condition. The *FT3 to FT4 ratio* has been found to be lower in LT4-treated patients with central hypothyroidism, compared to euthyroidism, questioning whether dose and/or modality (T4/T3 combination) of treatment could be improved [40].

Most patients with syndrome of *resistance to thyroid hormone*, but not all, are euthyroid and do not require treatment for hypothyroidism [41]. In euthyroid patients, LT4 treatment is used for other reasons, particularly to reduce the elevated TSH level to treat or prevent *goitre*.

Selective T4 resistance with normal T3 sensitivity is a rare condition, presumably caused by an unknown deiodinase type 2 defect, which becomes apparent only after thyroidectomy on LT4 monotherapy and requires additional LT3 substitution [42].

Both healthy thyroid hormone and TSH levels are genetically determined, and variation in their individual levels is limited, compared to that of the population [43–46]. In this respect, genes encoding the iodothyronine deiodinases were intensively studied because of their potential to alter the balance of thyroid hormones [47–49]. A preference for combined LT4/LT3 replacement therapy has been reported for hypothyroid patients with a distinct *polymorphisms* in the deiodinase type 2 gene (*rs225014*) and thyroid hormone transporter MCT10 (rs17606253) [47, 50]. However, treatment-relevant recommendations for specific genetic polymorphisms remain controversial and have not been worked out [51, 52].

A number of *influences* affect the required LT4 dose or necessitate a change of dose when they occur [30] (Table 11.1).

Table 11.1 Important influences on dose requirements of LT4 treatment

Factor	Influence
Sex	Modify influence is largely due to different lean weight.
Age	LT4 requirement is reduced with increasing age. Tolerance to the full dose may be lower in elderly patients, compared to younger patients, requiring more cautious dosing.
Body weight	LT4 requirement increases with increasing body weight.
Time of LT4 administration	Morning and evening medication is mostly equally effective.
Intake of food	In the fasting state, LT4 absorption rate is optimal. LT4 is recommended to be taken 30 min before breakfast.
Thyroid remnant	A complete loss of functional thyroid tissue results in FT3 instability. This may require an increase of LT4 dose or the addition of LT3.
Regulatory deficiencies	Equilibria between FT3, FT4 and TSH are altered on LT4 treatment, compared to thyroid health. TSH is impaired in secondary/tertiary hypothyroidism due to pituitary or hypothalamic disease.
Conversion efficiency	LT4 interferes with the activity of deiodinases type 1 and 2. Loss of the thyroid gland abolishes intra-thyroidal T4 to T3 conversion. Genetic polymorphisms in thyroid health and disease may affect T4 to T3 conversion rates.
Reduced sensitivity to thyroid hormone	Hereditary resistance syndromes or acquired resistance for instance due to interference of endocrine disruptors reduce the sensitivity to thyroid hormones. This results in compensated euthyroidism with different equilibria between TSH-FT4 and FT3 or may lead to hypothyroidism.
Disease aetiology	Athyreotic patients (e.g. due to thyroid cancer) tend to require higher doses of LT4. Conversion efficiency decreases due to the loss of TSH-FT3 feed-forward. In patients with autoimmune thyroiditis, TSH-FT3 feed-forward increases deiodinase activities. These diseases render FT3 concentrations non-proportional to those of FT4.
Pregnancy	LT4 dose requirements are increased due to an increased demand of thyroid hormones in pregnancy.
Comorbidity	Gastrointestinal absorption of thyroid hormones is reduced by prevalent gastrointestinal diseases, such as coeliac disease.
Use of other drugs	Many common drugs interfere with the absorption of LT4.
Adherence	Approx. 20% of patients do not adhere to regular LT4 use. Omission of a single dose is less influential due to the long plasma half-life of the drug.

11.2 Treatment Effects

The *success* of the treatment is to be evaluated according to clinical and biochemical criteria.

Some improvement in severe symptoms of hypothyroidism and an overall enhanced state of alertness and agility may be noticeable within days after commencing the medical treatment. More substantial improvement should be recognisable after 1–2 weeks. Achievement of complete symptomatic relief and a recovery back to "normal" should be expected to be a more gradual and prolonged process. It usually occurs over the course of several months. It is important to note that the restoration of clinical euthyroidism goes beyond the quantitative "normalisation" of thyroid hormones. It equally requires a reversal of the *structural change* in the many genomic actions and metabolic profile, both of which have been profoundly altered during the hypothyroid state, to permit a return to the previous healthy thyroidal state.

Quality of life (QoL) assessment may help inform on the general status of the treatment process, supporting the communication between patient and treating physician (Sect 7.9).

The *biochemical recovery* of the hypothyroid patient begins with measurable increases in serum FT4 and FT3 concentrations. This takes place within days and should in most patients bring the hormones up to their reference ranges within approx. 10 days. We note that after withdrawal of the LT4 drug, due to its long survival time in the circulation, a treatment effect could be felt for as long as 4 weeks. In contrast to FT4 and FT3 concentrations, which are fast to recover on LT4 treatment, the pituitary hormone TSH, due to dynamical compensation of the central components of the hypothalamic–pituitary–thyroid feedback control, requires a prolonged time of as much as 4–8 weeks to return to its reference range or settle on a new equilibrium after a change in LT4 dose. This means *measurements of TSH should be delayed* for approx. 2 months when commencing or changing LT4 treatment to achieve an equilibrated and obtain a reliable estimate. *Biochemical targets* include as an important treatment goal the restoration of the previously elevated TSH level into its reference range. TSH "normalisation" is regarded as a necessity for the success of the treatment in primary hypothyroidism. This alone is however not sufficient for many patients to achieve this goal and a satisfactory outcome. The *appropriate TSH level* requires individualised interpretation in context with the clinical presentation and the FT4 and FT3 concentrations that have been achieved with the treatment. We note that equilibria (working points) are frequently altered, compared to the previous healthy state.

In patients treated with a combination therapy of LT4 and LT3, the FT3 concentration is especially sensitive to pharmacokinetic effects due to its short half-life. In this subgroup, as well as in cases where there are doubts about the adequacy of hormone measurements for assessing the functional state, it may be useful to assess additional—not routinely measured—*biomarkers of thyroid hormone actions and signalling* (Sect. 10.3).

11.3 Issues and Controversies in the Treatment of Hypothyroidism

The current view on hypothyroidism and its treatment is dominated by the classical models, relying on a simplified subsystem of the greater hypothalamic–pituitary–thyroid system and concerning a limited perspective of FT4 physiology and its pituitary regulation by TSH [19, 31]. In contrast, recent insights, using among other investigations proof-of-concept mathematical modelling, have advanced our understanding of *the greater T3-inclusive system* of hypothalamic–pituitary–thyroid axis regulation (Chap. 5). The *new evidence* suggests that it is essential to consider an effective system regulation of the hypothalamic–pituitary–thyroid axis from a T3-inclusive perspective [6, 53, 54]. After all, T3 is the *chief biological thyroid hormone* and its homeostasis is critical to many bodily functions. The extended system incorporates FT3 homeostasis as a system goal. It thereby *integrates* the two main aspects of thyroid physiology, namely thyroid hormone production dominated by glandular T4 storage and supply and thyroid hormone demand and utilisation mainly mediated by T3 [55]. Thyroid regulation has been reviewed in detail in a dedicated Chap. 5. Briefly, preservation of a homeostatic level of FT3 is essential for efficiency in the performance of multiple T3-dependent reactions at an energetic optimum. Under circumstances when the previous homeostatic level becomes indefensible, it may be advantageous to adapt it to a new level. This *flexibility* to choose between the preservation of homeostasis and its adaptation supports optimum resilience in stressful situations. It *aligns the two concepts* of thyroid homeostasis and thyroid allostasis, rather than viewing them as different goals [9].

Since the classical hypothalamic–pituitary–thyroid model of TSH-FT4 regulation does not account for crucial properties of system regulation, we came to the conclusion that hypothalamic–pituitary–thyroid axis regulation needs *to include FT3 homeostasis*. This changes the perception of the roles of FT4 and TSH profoundly, from primary targets to relative contributors in supporting FT3 stability as long as possible in various adverse circumstances [54]. This view has also led to a novel clinical concept of *relational stability* (Chap. 2). The "classical" and new concepts have been contrasted in earlier chapters [54]. Here we examine the therapeutic implications.

Diagnostic and therapeutic goals can no longer be defined solely by the determination of TSH and the achievement of its "normalisation", but shift to *prioritise FT3 homeostasis* (Chap. 5). According to recent clinical studies, the latter is also more closely associated with patient symptom relief and prognostic outcome [56–58].

Hence, in *subclinical hypothyroidism*, the diagnostic distinction lies not so much in its formal classification as a disease, which is associated with a moderate TSH increase, but in the recognition of the multifaceted aetiology and differentiated interpretation of this laboratory constellation. The *treatment decision* hinges on whether corrective actions proactively driven by TSH are successful in preserving FT3 homeostasis. In the state of relational stability, each patient achieves a unique *personal and situational balance* (working point) between their FT3, FT4 and TSH levels [6]. Hence, as a *diagnostic imperative*, we must recognise the importance of personalised outcomes to avoid inappropriate generalisation and a one-size-fits-all approach [30, 59]. An advanced understanding of the regulatory mechanisms that are involved in thyroid hormone homeostasis, together with the predominance of presentation and the uniqueness of each patient's biochemistry (Fig. 10.1), provides an *opportunity for improved patient care*, particularly when the standard approach to treatment fails.

11.3.1 Treatment Failure

A substantial portion of hypothyroid patients *fails to achieve satisfactory relief of their symptoms* on standard treatment with LT4, despite successful "normalisation" of their TSH concentration [24, 28, 60–65]. On LT4 treatment, discrepancies frequently arise between biochemical euthyroidism, defined solely or predominantly by TSH measurement, and symptomatic clinical evaluation of euthyroidism, when residual hypothyroid symptoms persist despite an apparently "normal" TSH. Advances in our understanding of hypothalamic–pituitary–thyroid regulation may explain the discrepancy, having particularly demonstrated a *deficiency in normal TSH signalling* (loss of TSH feed-forward onto FT3) under these conditions (Chap. 5). *Instability in regulation* translates to variability in the biochemical response to LT4 therapy [66].

If a patient presents with persisting residual symptoms on standard LT4 treatment, *three situations* can be distinguished:

1. This patient may not yet have met the appropriate biochemical treatment targets.
2. The hypothyroid symptoms have not subsided despite the fact that standard biochemical targets have been reached and TSH "normalisation" was achieved.
3. Comorbidity with overlapping symptoms to hypothyroidism may be present or the psychological burden of a chronic disease may impair the patient's well-being.

As for the first issue, LT4 treatment may be considered *inefficient*, if it fails to "normalise" TSH concentration after 2 months. *Absorption tests* may help uncover any problems with inadequate drug absorption [67–69].

The second problem, the ineffectiveness of treatment in the face of apparently "normalised" TSH with LT4 is more challenging. A deeper understanding of the hypothalamic–pituitary–thyroid regulation and the consequences of *disruptive mechanisms*, such as deficient TSH signalling is required for explanation and possible correction [54]. As explained earlier, *disjoints* arise between the responses to exogenous LT4 administration of TSH and FT4, TSH and FT3, as well as FT3 and FT4, indicating different types of conversion failures or insensitivity syndromes, compared to the healthy state. Those can, at least partly, be viewed as an uncorrected, *persistent syndrome of low T3*. Consequently, these patients often fail to adequately respond to standard LT4 treatment and require additional LT3 substitution.

To address the third issue, symptomatic testing and case finding beyond thyroid examination is recommended (Fig. 10.5). A *broader evaluation* may include, among others, pituitary disease or related disease such as thyroid autoimmunity (thyroid peroxidase antibodies (TPO Ab), thyrogobulin antibodies (Tg Ab) and other diseases associated with thyroid autoimmune disease, such as adrenal insufficiency (hypocortisolism), pernicious anaemia (vitamin B12 deficiency), coeliac disease (gluten sensitivity), vitamin D deficiency and anaemia (ferritin, transferring saturation). In treated patients with hypothyroidism due to autoimmune thyroiditis, a subgroup of patients may suffer from autonomic and somatosensory dysfunction, leading to neuropathic symptoms and impaired QoL [70]. In autoimmune thyroiditis, the diversity of the gut microbiome and risk of bacterial overgrowth may be increased [71]. Quality of life questionnaires (ThyPRO scores) may help identify and discuss specific domains of patient concern.

We suggest a number of possible assessments and corrective actions in *a LT4-treatment refractory patient.*

1. Assess treatment adherence and query correct and regular use of medication [72].
2. Escalate LT4 dose by increments of 25–50 μg/day, unless the existing dose is already very large (>200 μg LT4/day).
3. Possibly divide the LT4 dose to two times a day (bid).
4. Prolong the interval of LT4 intake to meals and other potentially interfering drugs such as calcium preparations [73].
5. Switch the drug to another brand, because some commercial preparations are known to display less favourable pharmacological characteristics, compared to others.
6. Change the formulation of the medication from tablets to liquid, because the liquid formula improves the bioavailability of the drug [74, 75].
7. Opt for intravenous application of LT4 until biochemical normalisation has been achieved, because the long-lasting hypothyroid state may have impaired gastrointestinal absorption of the drug.
8. Perform a drug absorption test and test for the presence of a gastrointestinal disease associated with malabsorption, particularly coeliac disease, an autoimmune disorder occasionally associated with autoimmune thyroiditis [76].
9. Escalate LT4 dose aiming at lower TSH concentrations, close to its lower reference limit [35, 56].
10. Assess the relative responses of TSH and FT4 and their ratio to detect selective T4-resistance syndrome [77].
11. Assess the FT3 to FT4 ratio to uncover T4 to T3 conversion inefficiency/failure and potentially address this issue with additional LT3 substitution [26, 27, 66].
12. Examine shifts in the homeostatic equilibria between TSH, FT4 and FT3 and calculated parameters of thyroid hormone homeostasis (Chap. 5). Of note, TSH targets may be altered post-thyroidectomy [78, 79].
13. Use archived FT3 levels in thyroid health, when available, rather than TSH as a potential target for more rapid range-directed achievement of satisfactory treatment. Particularly in athyreotic patients, restoration of FT3 homeostasis should

take precedence over TSH normalisation from a regulatory perspective (Chaps. 2 and 5).

14. Assess and correct accompanying or overlapping symptoms with common non-thyroidal conditions including deficiencies in other hormones such as cortisol, minerals (e.g. iron deficiency) and vitamins (prevalent vitamin D and vitamin B deficiency syndromes) (Sect.11.7).

As discussed earlier, reconstruction of *personal working points* and the use of *calculated homeostatically derived functional parameters* provide additional tools for wider clinical exploration and testing [80–82]. The direct measurement of FT3 and the FT3 to FT4 ratio is a simple yet informative measure to uncover possible inefficiencies in the T4-converting process. Measurement of FT3 and SPINA-GD (see Sect. 10.3) is additionally useful for estimating global deiodinase activity, unless compromised by comorbidity leading to the low T3 syndrome. This strategy allows comparison of follow-up measurements with *archived markers* before the onset of disease whenever available [6]. *Alternative markers* of thyroid hormone actions and signalling may be situationally useful (Sect. 10.3).

In summary, although many patients do well on standard treatment, in a substantial proportion of patients, *residual hypothyroid symptoms persist* in the presence of a "normal" (within reference) TSH concentration. Identifiable *disjoints* in the expression of the respective equilibria between TSH, FT4 and FT3 are a common feature of many patients who do not adequately respond to or tolerate standard LT4 treatment. On the other hand, *over-treatment* must also be avoided by treatment monitoring, given the individual dosing requirements and a narrow range of tolerance of hormone substitution. Non-specific and *overlapping symptoms* with other diseases are also to be considered. A possible approach could use a *suggestive diagnostic and therapeutic algorithm* to the patient with persistent symptoms on standard therapy (Fig. 11.1). These patients require special and individualised care, including consideration of the therapeutic use of alternative drugs and LT3 medication.

11.4 Treatment Monitoring

Initially, symptomatic and biochemical *monitoring* is recommended at 2–4 week intervals to adjust the LT4 dose as needed. Once conditions have stabilised, half-yearly or yearly visits may suffice for routine testing, complemented by situational assessment in the event of the development of new or altered symptoms.

Measurement of serum TSH and FT4 concentrations is endorsed by guidelines, but measurement of FT3 is regarded as redundant. Our studies and experience disagree with this view. In our opinion, the *measurement of FT3* concentrations provides indispensable additional information into the important aspects of treatment success and failure (Chaps. 2 and 5). *Disrupted TSH signalling*, a progressive TSH-FT3 disjoint and T4 to T3 conversion inefficiencies have been a frequent

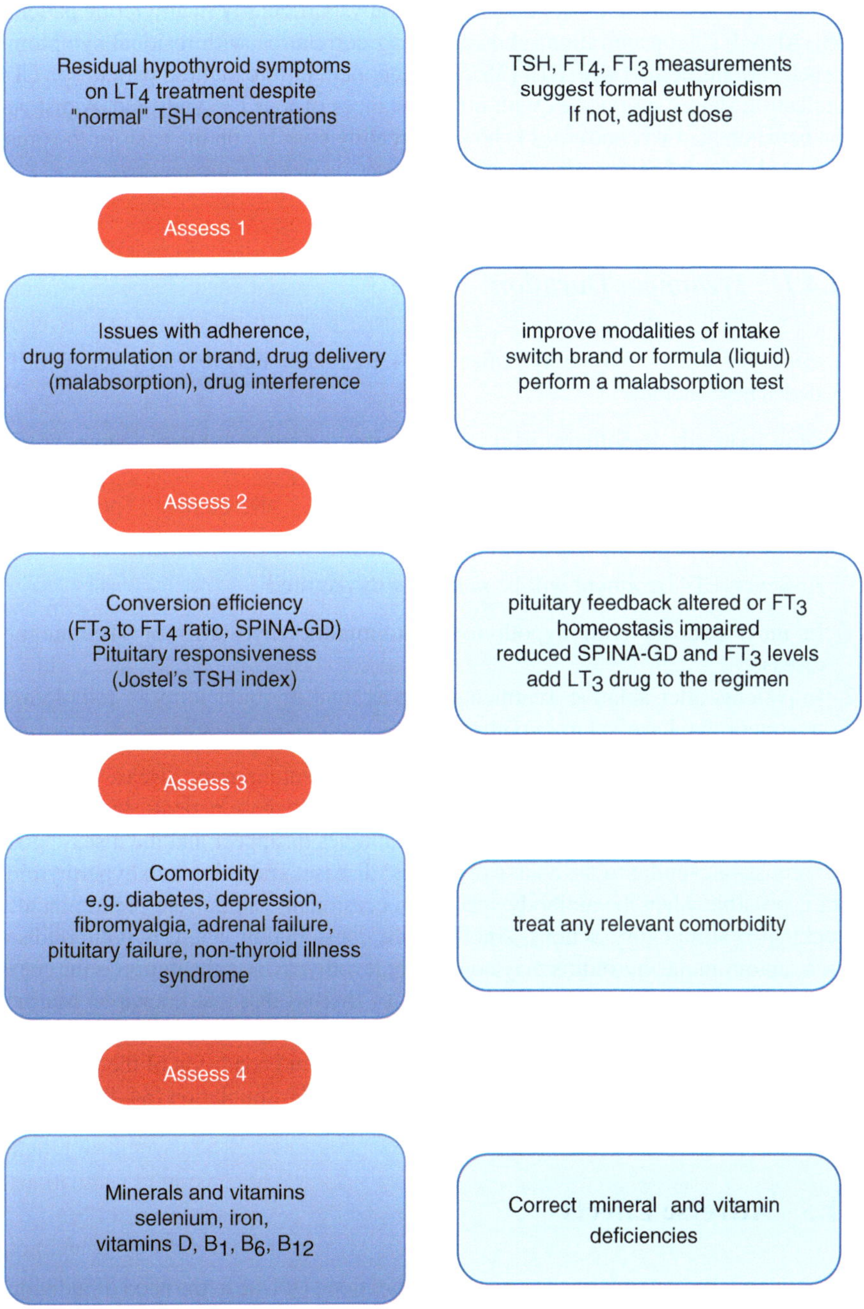

Fig. 11.1 A suggestive approach to the patient with persistent symptoms

finding in patients treated with LT4 monotherapy, particularly in athyreotic patients [66]. Also, FT3 concentrations showed strong correlation with residual symptoms in such patients treated with LT4 [35, 56]. Treatment failure in these patients on LT4 medication shares similarities with other instances of low T3 syndrome. A distinction between the two conditions is however readily possible on the basis of the presence or absence of severe non-thyroidal disease.

11.4.1 Treatment Duration

In *transient forms* of hypothyroidism, LT4 treatment may be only temporarily needed. These include

1. Drug-induced hypothyroidism (anti-thyroid drugs, lithium, amiodarone, interferon).
2. Non-autoimmune thyroiditis (deQuervain's thyroiditis, post-partum thyroiditis).

However, LT4 treatment will be *permanently* required

1. In most patients with hypothyroid autoimmune thyroiditis or Hashimoto's disease.
2. In patients after ablative treatments such as total thyroidectomy or radioiodine treatment that have led to hypothyroidism.

Notable exceptions are patients with hypothyroid autoimmune disease due to the action of TSH receptor (TSHR) blocking antibodies. In these patients, hypothyroidism may prove reversible if blocking type antibodies disappear and the disease goes into remission, similar to the course of Graves' disease. Transition into hyperthyroidism is possible when the antibody spectrum occasionally shifts from predominantly blocking to stimulatory actions. Another rare constellation where hypothyroidism due to autoimmune thyroiditis may not require levothyroxine substitution is the coexistence of a toxic adenoma—a combination of thyroid diseases known as Marine-Lenhart syndrome [83]. After hemithyroidectomy, patients may be able to avoid life-long LT4 substitution, depending on the amount and condition of the remaining tissue and its potential of regrowth upon moderate TSH stimulation [84–87].

11.5 Adverse Effects

LT4 is generally well tolerated as an oral medication [1]. Due to the need of individualised dose finding and a narrow range of tolerance of the hormone, *adverse effects* mainly arise from dosing error or dose inadequacy, with daily LT4 dosage being either too small or too large. This issue can readily be addressed by increasing or decreasing the LT4 dose as needed and subsequent retesting after a new equilibrium has been reached (4–8 weeks) [30]. Of note, the *optimum range* for individual dosing of the drug is narrow compared to the width of the interindividual reference range for FT4. This mirrors the personal working point of the homeostatic system (Fig. 10.1).

Over-treatment with thyroid hormones leads to a special form of hyperthyroidism, termed *thyrotoxicosis factitia*. Typical symptoms of overdosing include increased or irregular heartbeat, palpitations, nervousness and unrest. It is important to distinguish LT4-induced exogenous thyrotoxicosis from endogenous hyperthyroidism, as observed in Graves' disease or toxic adenomas. The former is accompanied by much lower FT3 concentrations, compared to the latter diseases, which diminishes the severity of the clinical syndrome [88, 89]. FT3 concentrations should therefore be determined in addition to TSH and FT4 measurements.

Allergic reactions to the natural hormone are extremely rare, but occasionally occur to components in the tablets other than the hormone. Allergy tests may help identify the cause. Tablets with different formulations are made available by some manufacturers upon request.

In patients with pre-existing coronary heart disease, owing to an *increase in oxygen demand* of the myocardium when transitioning from the hypothyroid to the euthyroid state, this condition may sometimes worsen. If cardiac symptoms develop or worsen, LT4 dose must first be reduced and then attempts should be made to increase it much more gradually and slowly than before. *Cardiac evaluation/intervention* may be needed prior to aiming for full substitution.

Possible interference with other medications has to be considered, among others, with coumarin anticoagulants, anti-diabetic drugs, antacids and calcium preparations [73]. The time interval between the intake of the thyroid medication and other drugs should then be extended to several hours.

In patients with *concomitant adrenal insufficiency* (Schmidt's syndrome) or pituitary deficiency (hypopituitarism), LT4 treatment must be delayed until after the cortisol deficiency has been treated and corrected. Otherwise, there is an increased risk that thyroid hormones could induce a potentially life-threatening exacerbation of these diseases (*Addisonian crisis*).

11.6 Treatment with Alternative Drugs

Although levothyroxine is generally considered safe and effective in the treatment of hypothyroidism and remains the guideline-endorsed standard of care, it does not meet the needs of many patients. *Alternative drugs have received renewed interest* and increased popularity among patients dissatisfied with the standard treatment. Among them are mainly LT3-containing drugs, such as *desiccated thyroid extracts* (DTE) of animal origin, which historically pre-dated the use of the synthetic LT4 drug, and *combinations of the synthetic hormones LT4 and LT3* [13, 16–18, 90–93].

New clinical trials were performed to compare the efficacy of DTE and LT4, which had not been initially conducted at the time when the shift from DTE to LT4 was made in the 1970s [17, 93–96]. It should be noted that the new preparations of thyroid extracts, unlike their historical counterparts, are far better standardised, using modern high pressure liquid chromatography (HPLC) techniques to maintain their content of thyroid hormones in different batches within United States Pharnacopeia (USP) specifications. In randomised controlled trials (RCTs), the statistical outcomes of DTE versus LT4-LT3 combination versus LT4 drugs for hypothyroid patients were similar [96]. Patient preference tended to favour the combination. In a cross-over design, the most symptomatic patients on LT4 responded positively to DTE and expressed their preference for combination treatment either as a synthetic drug or an extract. Despite the targeted increase in serum FT3 concentrations with the T3-containing drugs, no increase in adverse cardiovascular reactions was observed in those studies.

11.6.1 Desiccated Thyroid Hormone Extracts

Desiccated thyroid hormone extracts (DTEs) of porcine or bovine origin contain larger amounts of T3 than present in the human thyroid, with a T3 to T4 ratio of approximately 1:4. One grain (60 mg or 65 mg, depending on brand) of DTE contains about 38 μg of T4 and 9 μg of T3. Maintenance dosages of 60–120 mg DTE/day usually result in within-reference-range serum FT4 and FT3 levels [92]. The *pharmacodynamic equivalence* of T4 to T3 is estimated to be 3:1 [97]. This can be used to infer a reasonable dose estimate of DTE. However, patients may respond differently and further adjustments are absolutely required *on an individual basis* according to symptoms and biochemical tests. Serum FT3 levels tend to be temporarily increased when measured a few hours after the ingestion of DTE. Although clinical symptoms of thyrotoxicosis were not an issue in clinical studies, pharmacological short-term effects of transient hypertriiodothyroninaemia have not been sufficiently examined [93, 98–100]. If it is thought necessary, synthetic LT4 could be added to a slightly lower DTE dose to give a more physiological ratio of the two hormones for humans.

11.6.2 LT3/LT4 Combination Drugs

While DTE are most popular among American patients with hypothyroidism, *synthetic LT3/LT4 drugs* are more frequently used and approved as a prescription drug in some European countries.

Commercial drugs have been traditionally available in various strengths of LT3 (5, 10 or 20 μg) and LT4 (75, 100, 125 μg). In our view, the choice and dose combination should be guided by documenting and monitoring the improvement in measured serum FT3 concentrations to achieve symptomatic relief without clinical and biochemical T3 thyrotoxicosis. This approach best considers the physiological adaptivity of the natural TSH-controlled glandular T3 secretion and the consequences of its loss in athyreotic patients (Chap. 5). As a *safety measure*, FT3 concentrations are advised to be determined before and 3 h after the ingestion of the T3-containing drug to detect potentially "overshooting" *peak concentrations*.

The guideline issued by the European Thyroid Association provides some guidance when *switching* a patient from LT4 monotherapy to a combination of LT4 and LT3 [60]. Those are based on a randomized, double-blind, cross-over, pharmacodynamic equivalence study of LT4 and LT3 in ten thyroidectomized patients, which concluded that therapeutic substitution of LT3 for LT4 was achieved approximately at a 1:3 ratio [97].

The LT4 target dose in the combination z (μg/day) can be calculated according to the formula $z = x-3y$, where x = the TSH-normalising LT4 dose on LT4 monotherapy and y the target LT3 dose in the combination, which, in turn, is estimated with $y = x/17$ [60]. An online tool to perform these calculations has been made available by Dietrich [101, 102]. Further dose adjustments are then decided individually according to symptoms and biochemical markers.

The *pharmacological profile of LT3 drugs* is less favourable and less well studied, compared to that of LT4 drugs [98–100]. Any potential improvement such as the development of novel slow-release drugs has yet to reach marketability [103]. The biochemical responses to transient T3 spikes will be non-instantaneous and metabolically damped, making the true impact of such spikes less dangerous. Peak serum FT3 concentration can be measured 3 hours after drug intake.

In 18 clinical trials comparing combined therapy (LT4 + LT3) versus monotherapy (LT4) for adult patients with hypothyroidism, significant difference in *adverse events* were not found between the treatment modalities [23]. In a small short-term, double-blind RCT comparing LT4/LT3 combination with LT4/placebo in athyreotic patients with thyroid carcinoma, no adverse cardiovascular events were reported but a favourable change in diastolic function with the combination [104].

Fixed combinations in a drugs with fixed LT3 and LT4 combinations face challenges of different half-lives of the components, multiple daily dosing requirements for the T3 component and optimisation of the ratio of the components to be administered. When larger doses of T3 are required, their *divided administration* over at least two daily doses is recommended. Variable dosing of LT4 and LT3 as two separate individual drugs may further increase their adaptive use in some patients requiring more flexibility in dosing [30].

While the availability of limited safety data on LT3-containing drugs has to be acknowledged, staying on ineffective LT4 standard treatment may have its own unwanted consequences and risks for patients with persisting hypothyroid symptoms. For instance, data are lacking on long-term consequences and potential safety risks of a frequently observed increase in the FT4 to FT3 ratio in patients on LT4 monotherapy, even when their TSH is kept within the reference range and FT3 still remains below average. The elevated FT4 concentrations may not necessarily translate into toxic genomic T3 actions, because these indirect effects are dependent on T4 to T3 conversion which tends to be ineffective in this constellation [88].

However, T4 also exerts direct actions, not mediated by T3, when activating several *non-classical pathways* by binding to nuclear receptors via adaptor proteins (type 2 signalling), cytosolic receptors (type 3 signalling) and membrane-based receptors (type 4 signalling) [105] (see Sect. 3.2). Particularly, the *activation of the integrin receptor* by excess T4 concentrations is of concern because this pathway is *pro-oncogenic* and promotes the proliferation of cancer cells in vitro through its interaction with the αvß3 integrin receptor [106, 107]. These signalling types are differently controlled by T4 and T3, and the pituitary feedback loop on TSH is closed by type 1 signalling predominantly. Large epidemiological studies lend further support to a *possible link between LT4 treatment and cancer risk* [108, 109]. A cohort of the Swedish study population found an excess risk of different cancer types including breast, endometrium, other female genitals (ovaries not included), stomach, colon, liver, pancreas, urinary bladder, skin, leukaemia and unspecified primary tumour in association with LT4 treatment [110]. In a large retrospective Taiwanese case-control study, long-term LT4 use was significantly associated with an increased risk of brain, skin, pancreatic and breast cancers [111].

A *hormonal imbalance among various organs* may arise during LT4 monotherapy, as documented in animal studies [28, 112–114]. T3 tissue concentrations could be restored to their euthyroid levels in various organs by the administration of a combination of LT4 and LT3 to hypothyroid rodents, but not with LT4 alone [115]. These studies, although not performed in tissues of humans, do however suggest that disruptive mechanisms of the hypothalamic–pituitary–thyroid axis regulation have relevant treatment implications to warrant consideration (Chap. 5). Temperature differences between controlled primary hypothyroidism and healthy patients have been documented in humans [116].

11.6.3 Liothyronine Drugs

Liothyronine (LT3) drugs are commercially available. They have mainly been used *short term* in the preparation of patients for radioiodine treatment. After discontinuation of LT4 treatment in order to achieve a hypothyroid state with strongly elevated TSH levels (>20–30 mIU/l), which, in turn, promotes iodine uptake by the remaining thyrocytes, patients are temporally switched to LT3. The shorter half-life of the latter, compared to LT4, is advantageous in reducing the drug-free interval accompanied by unpleasant hypothyroid symptoms between withdrawal of medication and administration of radio iodine. The use of LT3 for this indication has declined since the introduction of recombinant human TSH as an alternative mode to stimulate radioiodine uptake for successful ablation of residual thyroid cancer cells after thyroidectomy [117]. Duration of LT3 usage in these hypothyroid patients is in the range of weeks, and the administered LT3 dose is approx. 3 × 20 μg/day.

Long-term use of LT3 monotherapy as an alternative to LT4 in the substitution therapy of hypothyroidism has been an exceptional option for a limited number of patients worldwide who either experienced no success of the standard treatment and T3/T4 combinations or were intolerant to it. This group of patients has not been well characterised—mutations in important pathways can only be suspected—but requires more attention and study. As discussed, pharmacodynamics was one of the main reasons to promote a shift to the LT4 drug in standard recommendations (Table 11.2).

Table 11.2 Comparison of the pharmacological properties of LT4 and LT3 drugs

Property	Levothyroxine drug (LT4)	Liothyronine drug (LT3)
Typical dose	1.6 μg/kg body weight/day However, the dose needs to be individually found and determined	Approx. 0.8 μg/kg body weight/day However, the dose needs to be individually found and determined
Dosing regime	Typically a single oral morning dose per day	To be divided in 2–3 daily doses
Bioavailability	70–80% of the orally given drug dose is absorbed in the small intestine in the fasting state Absorption rate is influenced by food, thyroid state, comorbidity and other drugs It can be much lower initially in severe hypothyroidism	Bioavailability is largely similar to that of T4
Peak concentration	Approx. 2 h after ingestion Delayed by food intake and by approx. 1 h in hypothyroid patients	Approx. 2–3 h after ingestion Delayed by food intake and in hypothyroid patients
Binding to transport proteins	Unbound, free fraction of FT4 is 0.02–0.03% Approx. 80% of circulating T4 is bound to TBG	Unbound, free fraction of FT3 is 0.2% T3 affinity for binding to proteins is 1/13 that of T4 Approx. 80% of circulating T3 are bound to TBG
Turn-over	Approx. 10%/day	Approx. 50–70%/day
Plasma half-life	Approx. 7 days, depending on thyroid function among other influences Approx. 1 day longer in hypothyroid patients	Approx. 1 day, depending on thyroid function, among other influences Longer in hypothyroid patients
Volume of distribution	12 l It tends to be larger (15 l) in hypothyroid patients	7—14 l Larger in hypothyroid patients
Clearance rate	0.055 l/h in euthyroid subjects 0.038 l/h in hypothyroid patients	2.7 l/h Reduced in hypothyroid patients
Transport into cells	T4 is actively transported into the cell across the plasma membrane by thyroid hormone transporters, such as OATP1A2, OATP1B1, OATP1C1, MCT8, etc. (Table 3.2) Transporters have different affinities for T4 and T3	T3 is actively transported into the cell across the plasma membrane by thyroid hormone transporters, such as OATP1A2, OATP1B1, OATP1C1, MCT8, etc. (Table 3.2) Transporters have different affinities for T4 and T3
Metabolism	The main metabolic route involves deiodination and conversion to either T3 or reverseT3, normally in a ratio of 1:1.	The metabolic route involves deiodination and conversion to 3,5-T2 and 3,3′-T2

For long-term FT3 use, a study over 17 years did not document increased clinical risks of atrial fibrillation, cardiovascular disease or fractures, compared to LT4 [118]. Antipsychotic co-medication was increased in patients taking LT3 [118]. Tariq and colleagues compared synthetic and natural LT3/LT4 combinations with LT4 and found no increase in risk with the prescription of the alternatives [95].

Although cardiovascular and skeletal risks of hyperthyroidism are well known, it should be emphasised that factitious thyrotoxicosis caused by LT4 overdose is an *entity of thyrotoxicosis entirely different from endogenous hyperthyroidism*. In clinical studies, the two conditions, displaying different equilibria, must not be aggregated and have to be analysed separately for the results to be informative on LT4 treatment [88, 89]. A failure to discriminate between subclinical and overt thyroid dysfunctions relates any study outcomes to the case mix rather than thyroid function. A lack of these important distinctions limits the information contributed by a plethora of studies measuring TSH only and reporting on associated cardiovascular or bone risks.

Of note, TSH measurement is not an accurate surrogate for FT3 determination, as has been documented for demographic characteristics including longevity [58].

11.7 Nutrition and Smoking

A link between *nutritional factors* and thyroid disease has long been recognised by ancient civilisations. *Severe iodine deficiency* has been a cause of hypothyroidism, particularly in newborns leading to cognitive deficits and the characteristic syndrome of cretinism [119]. *Mild iodine deficiency* is a prevalent cause of euthyroid goitre and thyroid nodular disease but does not lead to hypothyroidism (see Sect. 3.1).

In geographical regions where the native iodine content of most foods and beverages is low, adults can achieve sufficient iodine intake with the consumption of iodised salt (150–250 μg/d for adults). *Iodine fortification programmes* have greatly reduced the risk of iodine deficiency and thyroid dysfunction in Western populations. The iodine content and use of iodised salt may however vary across commercially available products, potentially introducing a risk to thyroid health. Pregnancy remains a period of increased susceptibility to iodine deficiency to warrant routine iodine supplementation. The therapeutic range of iodine is narrow, and *iodine excess* may also lead to iodine-induced hypothyroidism [120]. This is important for patients suffering from a thyroid autoimmune disease. They need to aim at a *balanced intake* to avoid both deficiency and excess. A frequently recommended dose for these patients is 100 μg/day of iodine, in case supplementation is deemed appropriate.

Selenium is another important trace element for thyroid health. Nutritional requirements were established even before deiodinases were identified as selenoenzymes. Apart from deiodinases, glutathione peroxidases (GPx) and thioredoxin reductases (TRx) also belong to the selenoenzyme family. They have strong antioxidant properties to protect thyroid cells from oxidative damage. In patients with autoimmune thyroiditis, selenium supplementation has been shown to mitigate the pathological immune response and decrease TPO Ab titers, potentially through raising plasma GPx activity and reducing hydrogen peroxide levels [121–128]. We note that selenium deficiency has also been implicated with increased thyroid cancer risk [129].

The diversity of the gut microbiome may also be altered in autoimmune thyroiditis [71].

Concentrations of iron, ferritin and vitamin D are frequently found to be low in patients with hypothyroidism. Vitamin B12 should also be tested, because it is occasionally associated with autoimmune thyroiditis. Since fatigue is one of the leading symptoms of these deficiencies shared with hypothyroidism, trace elements should be optimised. Furthermore, the *trace elements*, iodine, selenium, calcium, magnesium, zinc, iron, copper, nickel and vitamin D, are all associated with thyroid function and have been implicated to have immunomodulatory influences in autoimmune thyroiditis [126, 128, 130–138].

*Recommendations for target levels f*or 25-hydroxy vitamin D differ among various guidelines (50 ng/mL according to the Vitamin D council). Ferritin should be kept above 100 ng/mL and vitamin B12 should best be above 500 pg/mL.

Smoking impacts on the thyroid by increasing thiocyanate concentrations, an inhibitor of iodine uptake. Nicotine appears to have little, if any, thyroid-related effect. TSH levels appear to be slightly decreased in smokers, compared to non-smokers [131, 139–142]. Smoking does not predispose for hypothyroidism, but it may negatively influence the activity and course of the disease, accelerating the progression from latent to manifest autoimmune thyroiditis.

Among other endocrine organs, the function of the thyroid gland can be impaired by many widely used *endocrine-disrupting chemicals and nanoparticles* [143–147]. This includes clinically severe forms of acquired insensitivity to thyroid hormone and hypothyroidism (Sect. 6.6.1).

References

1. Biondi B, Wartofsky L. Treatment with thyroid hormone. Endocr Rev. 2014;35:433–512. https://doi.org/10.1210/er.2013-1083.
2. Chaker L, Bianco AC, Jonklaas J, Peeters RP. Hypothyroidism. Lancet. 2017;390:1550–62. https://doi.org/10.1016/S0140-6736(17)30703-1.
3. Hoermann R, Pekker MJ, Midgley JEM, Larisch R, Dietrich JW. Triiodothyronine secretion in early thyroid failure: the adaptive response of central feed-forward control. Eur J Clin Investig. 2020;50:e13192. https://doi.org/10.1111/eci.13192.
4. Galton VA, Schneider MJ, Clark AS, St Germain DL. Life without thyroxine to 3,5,3′-triiodothyronine conversion: studies in mice devoid of the 5′-deiodinases. Endocrinology. 2009;150:2957–63. https://doi.org/10.1210/en.2008-1572.
5. Ishii H, Inada M, Tanaka K, Mashio Y, Naito K, Nishikawa M, Matsuzuka F, Kuma K, Imura H. Induction of outer and inner ring monodeiodinases in human thyroid gland by thyrotropin. J Clin Endocrinol Metab. 1983;57:500–5. https://doi.org/10.1210/jcem-57-3-500.

6. Hoermann R, Midgley JEM, Larisch R, Dietrich JW. Relational stability in the expression of normality, variation, and control of thyroid function. Front Endocrinol (Lausanne). 2016;7:142. https://doi.org/10.3389/fendo.2016.00142.
7. Citterio CE, Veluswamy B, Morgan SJ, Galton VA, Banga JP, Atkins S, Morishita Y, Neumann S, Latif R, Gershengorn MC, Smith TJ, Arvan P. De novo triiodothyronine formation from thyrocytes activated by thyroid-stimulating hormone. J Biol Chem. 2017;292:15434–44. https://doi.org/10.1074/jbc.M117.784447.
8. Berberich J, Dietrich JW, Hoermann R, Müller MA. Mathematical modeling of the pituitary-thyroid feedback loop: role of a TSH-t3-shunt and sensitivity analysis. Front Endocrinol (Lausanne). 2018;9:91. https://doi.org/10.3389/fendo.2018.00091.
9. Hoermann R, Pekker M, Midgley JEM, Larisch R, Dietrich JW. Principles of endocrine regulation: reconciling tensions between robustness in performance and adaptation to change. Front Endocrinol (Lausanne). 2022;13:825107. https://doi.org/10.3389/fendo.2022.825107.
10. Hart Y, Antebi YE, Mayo AE, Friedman N, Alon U. Design principles of cell circuits with paradoxical components. Proc Natl Acad Sci USA. 2012;109:8346–51. https://doi.org/10.1073/pnas.1117475109.
11. Hoermann R, Midgley JEM, Larisch R, Dietrich JW. The role of functional thyroid capacity in pituitary thyroid feedback regulation. Eur J Clin Investig. 2018;48:e13003. https://doi.org/10.1111/eci.13003.
12. Lindholm J, Laurberg P. Hypothyroidism and thyroid substitution: historical aspects. J Thyroid Res. 2011;2011:809341. https://doi.org/10.4061/2011/809341.
13. Hennessey JV. Historical and current perspective in the use of thyroid extracts for the treatment of hypothyroidism. Endocr Pract. 2015;21:1161–70. https://doi.org/10.4158/EP14477.RA.
14. McAninch EA, Bianco AC. The history and future of treatment of hypothyroidism. Ann Intern Med. 2016;164:50–6. https://doi.org/10.7326/M15-1799.
15. Midgley JEM, Toft AD, Larisch R, Dietrich JW, Hoermann R. Time for a reassessment of the treatment of hypothyroidism. BMC Endocr Disord. 2019;19:37. https://doi.org/10.1186/s12902-019-0365-4.
16. Kahaly GJ, Gottwald-Hostalek U. Use of levothyroxine in the management of hypothyroidism: a historical perspective. Front Endocrinol (Lausanne). 2022;13:1054983. https://doi.org/10.3389/fendo.2022.1054983.
17. Idrees T, Palmer S, Maciel RMB, Bianco AC. Liothyronine and desiccated thyroid extract in the treatment of hypothyroidism. Thyroid. 2020;30:1399–413. https://doi.org/10.1089/thy.2020.0153.
18. Toloza FJK, Espinoza Suarez NR, El Kawkgi O, Golembiewski EH, Ponce OJ, Yao L, Maraka S, Singh Ospina NM, Brito JP. Patient experiences and perceptions associated with the use of desiccated thyroid extract. Medicina. 2020;56:161. https://doi.org/10.3390/medicina56040161.
19. Jonklaas J, Bianco AC, Bauer AJ, Burman KD, Cappola AR, Celi FS, Cooper DS, Kim BW, Peeters RP, Rosenthal MS, Sawka AM. Guidelines for the treatment of hypothyroidism: prepared by the American Thyroid Association task force on thyroid hormone replacement. Thyroid. 2014;24:1670–751. https://doi.org/10.1089/thy.2014.0028.
20. Grozinsky-Glasberg S, Fraser A, Nahshoni E, Weizman A, Leibovici L. Thyroxine-triiodothyronine combination therapy versus thyroxine monotherapy for clinical hypothyroidism: meta-analysis of randomized controlled trials. J Clin Endocrinol Metab. 2006;91:2592–9. https://doi.org/10.1210/jc.2006-0448.
21. Hennessey JV, Espaillat R. Current evidence for the treatment of hypothyroidism with levothyroxine/levotriiodothyronine combination therapy versus levothyroxine monotherapy. Int J Clin Pract. 2018;72:e13062–14. https://doi.org/10.1111/ijcp.13062.
22. Hoermann R, Midgley JEM, Larisch R, Dietrich JW. Lessons from randomised clinical trials for triiodothyronine treatment of hypothyroidism: have they achieved their objectives. J Thyroid Res. 2018;2018:3239197. https://doi.org/10.1155/2018/3239197.

23. Millan-Alanis JM, González-González JG, Flores-Rodríguez A, Singh Ospina N, Maraka S, Moreno-Peña PJ, Brito JP, González-Velázquez C, Rodríguez-Gutiérrez R. Benefits and harms of levothyroxine/l-triiodothyronine versus levothyroxine monotherapy for adult patients with hypothyroidism: systematic review and meta-analysis. Thyroid. 2021;31:1613–25. https://doi.org/10.1089/thy.2021.0270.
24. Peterson SJ, Cappola AR, Castro MR, Dayan CM, Farwell AP, Hennessey JV, Kopp PA, Ross DS, Samuels MH, Sawka AM, Taylor PN, Jonklaas J, Bianco AC. An online survey of hypothyroid patients demonstrates prominent dissatisfaction. Thyroid. 2018;28:707–21. https://doi.org/10.1089/thy.2017.0681.
25. Molewijk E, Fliers E, Dreijerink K, Van Dooren A, Heerdink R. Quality of life, daily functioning, and symptoms in hypothyroid patients on thyroid replacement therapy: a Dutch survey. J Clin Transl Endocrinol. 2024:100330. https://doi.org/10.1016/j.jcte.2024.100330.
26. Gullo D, Latina A, Frasca F, Le Moli R, Pellegriti G, Vigneri R. Levothyroxine monotherapy cannot guarantee euthyroidism in all athyreotic patients. PLoS One. 2011;6:e22552. https://doi.org/10.1371/journal.pone.0022552.
27. Hoermann R, Midgley JEM, Larisch R, Dietrich JW. Is pituitary TSH an adequate measure of thyroid hormone-controlled homoeostasis during thyroxine treatment. Eur J Endocrinol. 2013;168:271–80. https://doi.org/10.1530/EJE-12-0819.
28. McAninch EA, Bianco AC. New insights into the variable effectiveness of levothyroxine monotherapy for hypothyroidism. Lancet Diabetes Endocrinol. 2015;3:756–8. https://doi.org/10.1016/S2213-8587(15)00325-3.
29. Fitzgerald SP, Bean NG, Hennessey JV, Falhammar H. Thyroid testing paradigm switch from thyrotropin to thyroid hormones-future directions and opportunities in clinical medicine and research. Endocrine. 2021;74:285–9. https://doi.org/10.1007/s12020-021-02851-6.
30. Hoermann R, Midgley JEM, Larisch R, Dietrich JW. Individualised requirements for optimum treatment of hypothyroidism: complex needs, limited options. Drugs Context. 2019;8:212597. https://doi.org/10.7573/dic.212597.
31. Okosieme O, Gilbert J, Abraham P, Boelaert K, Dayan C, Gurnell M, Leese G, Mccabe C, Perros P, Smith V, Williams G, Vanderpump M. Management of primary hypothyroidism: statement by the British Thyroid Association executive committee. Clin Endocrinol. 2016;84:799–808. https://doi.org/10.1111/cen.12824.
32. Bianco AC, Dumitrescu A, Gereben B, Ribeiro MO, Fonseca TL, Fernandes GW, Bocco BMLC. Paradigms of dynamic control of thyroid hormone signaling. Endocr Rev. 2019;40:1000–47. https://doi.org/10.1210/er.2018-00275.
33. Jonklaas J, Bianco AC, Cappola AR, Celi FS, Fliers E, Heuer H, Mcaninch EA, Moeller LC, Nygaard B, Sawka AM, Watt T, Dayan CM. Evidence-based use of levothyroxine/liothyronine combinations in treating hypothyroidism: a consensus document. Thyroid. 2021;31:156–82. https://doi.org/10.1089/thy.2020.0720.
34. Brigante G, Santi D, Boselli G, Margiotta G, Corleto R, Monzani ML, Craparo A, Locaso M, Sperduti S, Roy N, Casarini L, Trenti T, Tagliavini S, De Santis MC, Roli L, Rochira V, Simoni M. Randomized double-blind placebo-controlled trial on levothyroxine and liothyronine combination therapy in totally thyroidectomized subjects: the Levolio study. Eur J Endocrinol. 2024;190:12–22. https://doi.org/10.1093/ejendo/lvad172.
35. Hoermann R, Midgley JEM, Larisch R, Dietrich JW. Functional and symptomatic individuality in the response to levothyroxine treatment. Front Endocrinol (Lausanne). 2019;10:664. https://doi.org/10.3389/fendo.2019.00664.
36. Colucci P, Yue CS, Ducharme M, Benvenga S. A review of the pharmacokinetics of levothyroxine for the treatment of hypothyroidism. Eur Endocrinol. 2013;9:40–7. https://doi.org/10.17925/EE.2013.09.01.40.
37. Rajput R, Chatterjee S, Rajput M. Can levothyroxine be taken as evening dose? Comparative evaluation of morning versus evening dose of levothyroxine in treatment of hypothyroidism. J Thyroid Res. 2011;2011:1–5. https://doi.org/10.4061/2011/505239.

38. Ehrenkranz J, Bach PR, Snow GL, Schneider A, Lee JL, Ilstrup S, Bennett ST, Benvenga S. Circadian and circannual rhythms in thyroid hormones: determining the TSH and free T4 reference intervals based upon time of day, age, and sex. Thyroid. 2015;25:954–61. https://doi.org/10.1089/thy.2014.0589.
39. Wall CR. Myxedema coma: diagnosis and treatment. Am Fam Physician. 2000;62:2485–90.
40. Sesmilo G, Simó O, Choque L, Casamitjana R, Puig-Domingo M, Halperin I. Serum free triiodothyronine (t3) to free thyroxine (t4) ratio in treated central hypothyroidism compared with primary hypothyroidism and euthyroidism. Endocrinol Nutr. 2011;58:9–15. https://doi.org/10.1016/j.endonu.2010.09.006.
41. Pappa T, Refetoff S. Resistance to thyroid hormone beta: a focused review. Front Endocrinol (Lausanne). 2021;12:656551. https://doi.org/10.3389/fendo.2021.656551.
42. Lacámara N, Lecumberri B, Barquiel B, Escribano A, González-Casado I, Álvarez-Escolá C, Aleixandre-Blanquer F, Morales F, Alfayate R, Bernal-Soriano MC, Miralles R, Yildirim Simsir I, Özgen AG, Bernal J, Berbel P, Moreno JC. Identification of resistance to exogenous thyroxine in humans. Thyroid. 2020;30:1732–44. https://doi.org/10.1089/thy.2019.0825.
43. Hansen PS, Brix TH, Sørensen TIA, Kyvik KO, Hegedüs L. Major genetic influence on the regulation of the pituitary-thyroid axis: a study of healthy Danish twins. J Clin Endocrinol Metab. 2004;89:1181–7. https://doi.org/10.1210/jc.2003-031641.
44. Panicker V, Wilson SG, Spector TD, Brown SJ, Falchi M, Richards JB, Surdulescu GL, Lim EM, Fletcher SJ, Walsh JP. Heritability of serum TSH, free T4 and free T3 concentrations: a study of a large UK twin cohort. Clin Endocrinol. 2008;68:652–9. https://doi.org/10.1111/j.1365-2265.2007.03079.x.
45. Andersen S, Pedersen KM, Bruun NH, Laurberg P. Narrow individual variations in serum T4 and T3 in normal subjects: a clue to the understanding of subclinical thyroid disease. J Clin Endocrinol Metab. 2002;87:1068–72. https://doi.org/10.1210/jcem.87.3.8165.
46. Lightman SL. Clinical endocrinology-time for a reset. J Endocr Soc. 2024;8:bvae024. https://doi.org/10.1210/jendso/bvae024.
47. Panicker V, Cluett C, Shields B, Murray A, Parnell KS, Perry JRB, Weedon MN, Singleton A, Hernandez D, Evans J, Durant C, Ferrucci L, Melzer D, Saravanan P, Visser TJ, Ceresini G, Hattersley AT, Vaidya B, Dayan CM, Frayling TM. A common variation in deiodinase 1 gene dio1 is associated with the relative levels of free thyroxine and triiodothyronine. J Clin Endocrinol Metab. 2008;93:3075–81. https://doi.org/10.1210/jc.2008-0397.
48. Taylor PN, Panicker V, Sayers A, Shields B, Iqbal A, Bremner AP, Beilby JP, Leedman PJ, Hattersley AT, Vaidya B, Frayling T, Evans J, Tobias JH, Timpson NJ, Walsh JP, Dayan CM. A meta-analysis of the associations between common variation in the pde8b gene and thyroid hormone parameters, including assessment of longitudinal stability of associations over time and effect of thyroid hormone replacement. Eur J Endocrinol. 2011;164:773–80. https://doi.org/10.1530/EJE-10-0938.
49. Bianco AC, Kim BS. Pathophysiological relevance of deiodinase polymorphism. Curr Opin Endocrinol Diabetes Obes. 2018;25:341–6. https://doi.org/10.1097/MED.0000000000000428.
50. Carlé A, Faber J, Steffensen R, Laurberg P, Nygaard B. Hypothyroid patients encoding combined MCT10 and dio2 gene polymorphisms may prefer L-T3 + L-T4 combination treatment—data using a blind, randomized, clinical study. Eur Thyroid J. 2017;6:143–51. https://doi.org/10.1159/000469709.
51. Deng Y, Han Y, Gao S, Dong W, Yu Y. The physiological functions and polymorphisms of type ii deiodinase. Endocrinol Metab (Seoul). 2023;38:190–202. https://doi.org/10.3803/EnM.2022.1599.
52. Jensen CZ, Isaksen JL, Ahlberg G, Olesen MS, Nygaard B, Ellervik C, Kanters JK. Association of dio2 and MCT10 polymorphisms with persistent symptoms in LT4-treated patients in the UK biobank. J Clin Endocrinol Metab. 2024;109:e613–22. https://doi.org/10.1210/clinem/dgad556.

53. Hoermann R, Midgley JEM, Larisch R, Dietrich JW. Advances in applied homeostatic modelling of the relationship between thyrotropin and free thyroxine. PLoS One. 2017;12:e0187232. https://doi.org/10.1371/journal.pone.0187232.
54. Hoermann R, Pekker MJ, Midgley JEM, Dietrich JW. The role of supporting and disruptive mechanisms of FT3 homeostasis in regulating the hypothalamic-pituitary-thyroid axis. Ther Adv Endocrinol Metab. 2023;14:20420188231158163. https://doi.org/10.1177/20420188231158163.
55. Hoermann R, Midgley JEM, Larisch R, Dietrich JW. Integration of peripheral and glandular regulation of triiodothyronine production by thyrotropin in untreated and thyroxine-treated subjects. Horm Metab Res. 2015;47:674–80. https://doi.org/10.1055/s-0034-1398616.
56. Larisch R, Midgley JEM, Dietrich JW, Hoermann R. Symptomatic relief is related to serum free triiodothyronine concentrations during follow-up in levothyroxine-treated patients with differentiated thyroid cancer. Exp Clin Endocrinol Diabetes. 2018;126:546–52. https://doi.org/10.1055/s-0043-125064.
57. Fitzgerald SP, Bean NG, Falhammar H, Tuke J. Clinical parameters are more likely to be associated with thyroid hormone levels than with thyrotropin levels: a systematic review and meta-analysis. Thyroid. 2020;30:1695–709. https://doi.org/10.1089/thy.2019.0535.
58. Lawton RI, Sabatini BL, Hochbaum DR. Longevity, demographic characteristics, and socio-economic status are linked to triiodothyronine levels in the general population. Proc Natl Acad Sci USA. 2024;121(2):e2308652121. https://doi.org/10.1073/pnas.2308652121.
59. Fisher AJ, Medaglia JD, Jeronimus BF. Lack of group-to-individual generalizability is a threat to human subjects research. Proc Natl Acad Sci USA. 2018;115:E6106–15. https://doi.org/10.1073/pnas.1711978115.
60. Wiersinga WM, Duntas L, Fadeyev V, Nygaard B, Vanderpump MP. 2012 ETA guidelines: the use of L-T4 + L-T3 in the treatment of hypothyroidism. Eur Thyroid J. 2012;1:55–71. https://doi.org/10.1159/000339444.
61. Wiersinga WM. Paradigm shifts in thyroid hormone replacement therapies for hypothyroidism. Nat Rev Endocrinol. 2014;10:164–74. https://doi.org/10.1038/nrendo.2013.258.
62. Winther KH, Cramon P, Watt T, Bjorner JB, Ekholm O, Feldt-Rasmussen U, Groenvold M, Rasmussen ÅK, Hegedüs L, Bonnema SJ. Disease-specific as well as generic quality of life is widely impacted in autoimmune hypothyroidism and improves during the first six months of levothyroxine therapy. PLoS One. 2016;11:e0156925. https://doi.org/10.1371/journal.pone.0156925.
63. Biondi B, Celi FS, Mcaninch EA. Critical approach to hypothyroid patients with persistent symptoms. J Clin Endocrinol Metab. 2023;108:2708–16. https://doi.org/10.1210/clinem/dgad224.
64. Hidalgo J, Vallejo BA, Soto Jacome C, Ayala IN, Cordova S, Duran M, Golembiewski E, Toro-Tobon D, Brito JP. Real practice assessment of persistent symptoms after initiation of levothyroxine. Endocr Pract. 2024;30:95–100. https://doi.org/10.1016/j.eprac.2023.10.132.
65. Łukawska-Tatarczuk M, Franek E. Causes of difficulties with adequate levothyroxine substitution—an immunoendocrine perspective. Endokrynol Pol. 2024; https://doi.org/10.5603/ep.100034.
66. Midgley JEM, Larisch R, Dietrich JW, Hoermann R. Variation in the biochemical response to L-thyroxine therapy and relationship with peripheral thyroid hormone conversion efficiency. Endocr Connect. 2015;4:196–205. https://doi.org/10.1530/EC-15-0056.
67. Walker JN, Shillo P, Ibbotson V, Vincent A, Karavitaki N, Weetman AP, Wass JAH, Allahabadia A. A thyroxine absorption test followed by weekly thyroxine administration: a method to assess non-adherence to treatment. Eur J Endocrinol. 2013;168:913–7. https://doi.org/10.1530/EJE-12-1035.
68. Robertson HMA, Narayanaswamy AKP, Pereira O, Copland SA, Herriot R, Mckinlay AW, Bevan JS, Abraham P. Factors contributing to high levothyroxine doses in primary hypothyroidism: an interventional audit of a large community database. Thyroid. 2014;24:1765–71. https://doi.org/10.1089/thy.2013.0661.

69. Müssig K. Levothyroxine absorption test—an underused tool. Exp Clin Endocrinol Diabetes. 2023;131:629–30. https://doi.org/10.1055/a-2210-1109.
70. Bazika-Gerasch B, Kumowski N, Enax-Krumova E, Kaisler M, Eitner LB, Maier C, Dietrich JW. Impaired autonomic function and somatosensory disturbance in patients with treated autoimmune thyroiditis. Sci Rep. 2024;14:12358. https://doi.org/10.1038/s41598-024-63158-w.
71. Alkader DAA, Asadi N, Solangi U, Singh R, Rasuli SF, Farooq MJ, Raheela FNU, Waseem R, Gilani SM, Abbas K, Ahmed M, Tanoh DB, Shah HH, Dulal A, Hussain MS, Talpur AS. Exploring the role of gut microbiota in autoimmune thyroid disorders: a systematic review and meta-analysis. Front Endocrinol (Lausanne). 2023;14:1238146. https://doi.org/10.3389/fendo.2023.1238146.
72. Cappelli C, Castello R, Marini F, Paoletta A, Marchetti M, Saullo M, Cristiano A, Pirola I, Gandossi E, Ferlin A, Castellano M. Adherence to levothyroxine treatment among patients with hypothyroidism: a northeastern Italian survey. Front Endocrinol (Lausanne). 2018;9:699. https://doi.org/10.3389/fendo.2018.00699.
73. Benvenga S. L-T4 therapy in the presence of pharmacological interferents. Front Endocrinol (Lausanne). 2020;11:607446. https://doi.org/10.3389/fendo.2020.607446.
74. Fallahi P, Ferrari SM, Ruffilli I, Ragusa F, Biricotti M, Materazzi G, Miccoli P, Antonelli A. Advancements in the treatment of hypothyroidism with L-T4 liquid formulation or soft gel capsule: an update. Expert Opin Drug Deliv. 2017;14:647–55. https://doi.org/10.1080/17425247.2016.1227782.
75. Liu H, Li W, Zhang W, Sun S, Chen C. Levothyroxine: conventional and novel drug delivery formulations. Endocr Rev. 2023;44:393–416. https://doi.org/10.1210/endrev/bnac030.
76. Virili C, Antonelli A, Santaguida MG, Benvenga S, Centanni M. Gastrointestinal malabsorption of thyroxine. Endocr Rev. 2019;40:118–36. https://doi.org/10.1210/er.2018-00168.
77. Laclaustra M, Moreno-Franco B, Lou-Bonafonte JM, Mateo-Gallego R, Casasnovas JA, Guallar-Castillon P, Cenarro A, Civeira F. Impaired sensitivity to thyroid hormones is associated with diabetes and metabolic syndrome. Diabetes Care. 2019;42:303–10. https://doi.org/10.2337/dc18-1410.
78. Ito M, Miyauchi A, Morita S, Kudo T, Nishihara E, Kihara M, Takamura Y, Ito Y, Kobayashi K, Miya A, Kubota S, Amino N. TSH-suppressive doses of levothyroxine are required to achieve preoperative native serum triiodothyronine levels in patients who have undergone total thyroidectomy. Eur J Endocrinol. 2012;167:373–8. https://doi.org/10.1530/EJE-11-1029.
79. Ito M, Miyauchi A, Hisakado M, Yoshioka W, Ide A, Kudo T, Nishihara E, Kihara M, Ito Y, Kobayashi K, Miya A, Fukata S, Nishikawa M, Nakamura H, Amino N. Biochemical markers reflecting thyroid function in athyreotic patients on levothyroxine monotherapy. Thyroid. 2017;27:484–90. https://doi.org/10.1089/thy.2016.0426.
80. Leow MKS, Goede SL. The homeostatic set point of the hypothalamus-pituitary-thyroid axis—maximum curvature theory for personalized euthyroid targets. Theor Biol Med Model. 2014;11:35. https://doi.org/10.1186/1742-4682-11-35.
81. Goede SL, Leow MKS, Smit JW, Dietrich JW. A novel minimal mathematical model of the hypothalamus-pituitary-thyroid axis validated for individualized clinical applications. Math Biosci. 2014;249:1–7. https://doi.org/10.1016/j.mbs.2014.01.001.
82. Dietrich JW, Landgrafe-Mende G, Wiora E, Chatzitomaris A, Klein HH, Midgley JEM, Hoermann R. Calculated parameters of thyroid homeostasis: emerging tools for differential diagnosis and clinical research. Front Endocrinol (Lausanne). 2016;7:57. https://doi.org/10.3389/fendo.2016.00057.
83. Mathiopoulou M, Engel-Bicik I. Hyperthyroidism in 2 forms: the Marine-Lenhart syndrome. Endocr Abstr. 2023; https://doi.org/10.1530/endoabs.93.OC42.
84. Ito M, Miyauchi A, Kang S, Hisakado M, Yoshioka W, Ide A, Kudo T, Nishihara E, Kihara M, Ito Y, Kobayashi K, Miya A, Fukata S, Nakamura H, Amino N. Effect of the presence of remnant thyroid tissue on the serum thyroid hormone balance in thyroidectomized patients. Eur J Endocrinol. 2015;173:333–40. https://doi.org/10.1530/EJE-15-0138.

85. Ahn D, Sohn JH, Jeon JH. Hypothyroidism following hemithyroidectomy: incidence, risk factors, and clinical characteristics. J Clin Endocrinol Metab. 2016;101:1429–36. https://doi.org/10.1210/jc.2015-3997.
86. Park S, Jeon MJ, Song E, Oh H-S, Kim M, Kwon H, Kim TY, Hong SJ, Shong YK, Kim WB, Sung T-Y, Kim WG. Clinical features of early and late postoperative hypothyroidism after lobectomy. J Clin Endocrinol Metab. 2017;102:1317–24. https://doi.org/10.1210/jc.2016-3597.
87. Yaniv D, Vainer I, Amir I, Robenshtok E, Hirsch D, Watt T, Hilly O, Shkedy Y, Shpitzer T, Bachar G. Quality of life following lobectomy versus total thyroidectomy is significantly related to hypothyroidism. J Surg Oncol. 2022;126:640–8. https://doi.org/10.1002/jso.26983.
88. Hoermann R, Midgley JEM, Larisch R, Dietrich JW. Heterogenous biochemical expression of hormone activity in subclinical/overt hyperthyroidism and exogenous thyrotoxicosis. J Clin Transl Endocrinol. 2020;19:100219. https://doi.org/10.1016/j.jcte.2020.100219.
89. Deguchi-Horiuchi H, Ito M, Takahashi S, Kousaka K, Hisakado M, Fukata S, Kudo T, Nishihara E, Nishikawa M, Miyauchi A, Akamizu T. Comparison of pathophysiology in subclinical hyperthyroidism with different etiologies. Endocr J. 2024; https://doi.org/10.1507/endocrj.EJ23-0497.
90. Hughes DA, Skiadas K, Fitzsimmons D, Anderson P, Heald A. Liothyronine for hypothyroidism: a candidate for disinvestment or in need of further research? A value of information analysis. BMJ Open. 2021;11:e051702. https://doi.org/10.1136/bmjopen-2021-051702.
91. Ettleson MD, Ibarra S, Wan W, Peterson S, Laiteerapong N, Bianco AC. Demographic, healthcare access, and dietary factors associated with thyroid hormone treatments for hypothyroidism. J Clin Endocrinol Metab. 2023;108:e1614–23. https://doi.org/10.1210/clinem/dgad331.
92. Heald A, Taylor PN, Premawardhana LD, Stedman M, Dayan CM. Natural desiccated thyroid for the treatment of hypothyroidism. Front Endocrinol (Lausanne). 2024;14:1309159. https://doi.org/10.3389/fendo.2023.1309159/full.
93. Riis KR, Larsen CB, Bonnema SJ. Potential risks and benefits of desiccated thyroid extract for the treatment of hypothyroidism: a systematic review. Thyroid. 2024; https://doi.org/10.1089/thy.2023.0649.
94. Hoang TD, Olsen CH, Mai VQ, Clyde PW, Shakir MK. Desiccated thyroid extract compared with levothyroxine in the treatment of hypothyroidism: a randomized, double-blind, crossover study. J Clin Endocrinol Metab. 2013;98:1982–90. https://doi.org/10.1210/jc.2012-4107.
95. Tariq A, Wert Y, Cheriyath P, Joshi R. Effects of long-term combination LT4 and LT3 therapy for improving hypothyroidism and overall quality of life. South Med J. 2018;111:363–9. https://doi.org/10.14423/SMJ.0000000000000823.
96. Shakir MKM, Brooks DI, Mcaninch EA, Fonseca TL, Mai VQ, Bianco AC, Hoang TD. Comparative effectiveness of levothyroxine, desiccated thyroid extract, and levothyroxine+liothyronine in hypothyroidism. J Clin Endocrinol Metab. 2021;106:e4400–13. https://doi.org/10.1210/clinem/dgab478.
97. Celi FS, Zemskova M, Linderman JD, Babar NI, Skarulis MC, Csako G, Wesley R, Costello R, Penzak SR, Pucino F. The pharmacodynamic equivalence of levothyroxine and liothyronine: a randomized, double blind, cross-over study in thyroidectomized patients. Clin Endocrinol. 2010;72:709–15. https://doi.org/10.1111/j.1365-2265.2009.03700.x.
98. Jonklaas J, Burman KD, Wang H, Latham KR. Single-dose T3 administration: kinetics and effects on biochemical and physiological parameters. Ther Drug Monit. 2015;37:110–8. https://doi.org/10.1097/FTD.0000000000000113.
99. Jonklaas J, Burman KD. Daily administration of short-acting liothyronine is associated with significant triiodothyronine excursions and fails to alter thyroid-responsive parameters. Thyroid. 2016;26:770–8. https://doi.org/10.1089/thy.2015.0629.
100. Goede SL, Latham KR, Leow MKS, Jonklaas J. High resolution free triiodothyronine-thyrotropin (ft3-tsh) responses to a single oral dose of liothyronine in humans: evidence of distinct inter-individual differences unraveled using an electrical network model. J Biol Syst. 2017;25:119–43. https://doi.org/10.1142/S0218339017500073.

101. Dietrich JW. Calculator software helping to determine L-T4 and L-T3 substitution dosage according to the algorithms provided by the European Thyroid Association (ETA). Source. 2022; https://doi.org/10.5281/zenodo.5720631.
102. Dietrich JW. Triangolo (1.0). zenodo. 2022; https://doi.org/10.5281/zenodo.5720632.
103. Idrees T, Price J, Piccariello T, Bianco AC. Sustained release T3 therapy: animal models and translational applications. Front Endocrinol (Lausanne). 2019;10:544.
104. Biondi B, Pucci M, Pontieri G, Formisano P, Esposito R. Preliminary results of a double-blind randomized controlled trial evaluating the cardiometabolic effects of levothyroxine and liothyronine compared to levothyroxine with placebo in athyreotic low-risk thyroid cancer patients. Thyroid. 2023;33:1402–13. https://doi.org/10.1089/thy.2023.0135.
105. Flamant F, Cheng SY, Hollenberg AN, Moeller LC, Samarut J, Wondisford FE, Yen PM, Refetoff S. Thyroid hormone signaling pathways: time for a more precise nomenclature. Endocrinology. 2017;158:2052–7. https://doi.org/10.1210/en.2017-00250.
106. Davis PJ, Tang HY, Hercbergs A, Lin HY, Keating KA, Mousa SA. Bioactivity of thyroid hormone analogs at cancer cells. Front Endocrinol (Lausanne). 2018;9:739. https://doi.org/10.3389/fendo.2018.00739.
107. Hercbergs A. Clinical implications and impact of discovery of the thyroid hormone receptor on integrin αvβ3—a review. Front Endocrinol (Lausanne). 2019;10:565. https://doi.org/10.3389/fendo.2019.00565.
108. Hellevik AI, Asvold BO, Bjøro T, Romundstad PR, Nilsen TIL, Vatten LJ. Thyroid function and cancer risk: a prospective population study. Cancer Epidemiol Biomarkers Prev. 2009;18:570–4. https://doi.org/10.1158/1055-9965.EPI-08-0911.
109. Kim MS, Lee JW, Hyun MK, Song YS. Risk of subsequent primary cancers in thyroid cancer survivors according to the dose of levothyroxine: a nationwide cohort study. Endocrinol Metab (Seoul). 2024;39:288–99. https://doi.org/10.3803/EnM.2023.1815.
110. Wändell P, Carlsson AC, Li X, Sundquist J, Sundquist K. Levothyroxine treatment is associated with an increased relative risk of overall and organ specific incident cancers—a cohort study of the Swedish population. Cancer Epidemiol. 2020;66:101707. https://doi.org/10.1016/j.canep.2020.101707.
111. Wu CC, Islam MM, Nguyen PA, Poly TN, Wang CH, Iqbal U, Li YJ, Yang HC. Risk of cancer in long-term levothyroxine users: retrospective population-based study. Cancer Sci. 2021;112:2533–41. https://doi.org/10.1111/cas.14908.
112. Escobar-Morreale HF, Obregón MJ, Escobar Del Rey F, Morereale De Escobar G. Replacement therapy for hypothyroidism with thyroxine alone does not ensure euthyroidism in all tissues, as studied in thyroidectomized rats. J Clin Invest. 1995;96:2828–38. https://doi.org/10.1172/JCI118353.
113. Werneck De Castro JP, Fonseca TL, Ueta CB, Mcaninch EA, Abdalla SM, Wittmann G, Lechan RM, Gereben B, Bianco AC. Differences in hypothalamic type 2 deiodinase ubiquitination explain localized sensitivity to thyroxine. J Clin Invest. 2015;125:769–81. https://doi.org/10.1172/JCI77588.
114. Dietrich JW, Midgley JEM, Larisch R, Hoermann R. Of rats and men: thyroid homeostasis in rodents and human beings. Lancet Diabetes Endocrinol. 2015;3:932–3. https://doi.org/10.1016/S2213-8587(15)00421-0.
115. Escobar-Morreale HF, Del Rey FE, Obregón MJ, De Escobar GM. Only the combined treatment with thyroxine and triiodothyronine ensures euthyroidism in all tissues of the thyroidectomized rat. Endocrinology. 1996;137:2490–502. https://doi.org/10.1210/endo.137.6.8641203.
116. Romero-Ibarguengoitia ME, Garza-Silva A, Rivera-Cavazos A, Morales-Rodriguez DP, González-Peña OI, Barco-Flores IA, Manilla-Muñoz E, Villarreal-Leal E, González-Cantú A. Temperature differences between controlled primary hypothyroidism and healthy patients: an exploratory study. J Endocr Soc. 2024;8:bvad175. https://doi.org/10.1210/jendso/bvad175.
117. Schlumberger M, Leboulleux S. Current practice in patients with differentiated thyroid cancer. Nat Rev Endocrinol. 2021;17:176–88. https://doi.org/10.1038/s41574-020-00448-z.

118. Leese GP, Soto-Pedre E, Donnelly LA. Liothyronine use in a 17 year observational population-based study—the TEARS study. Clin Endocrinol. 2016;85:918–25. https://doi.org/10.1111/cen.13052.
119. Zimmermann MB, Jooste PL, Pandav CS. Iodine-deficiency disorders. Lancet. 2008;372:1251–62. https://doi.org/10.1016/S0140-6736(08)61005-3.
120. Fan X, Zhao L, Wang S, Song K, Wang B, Xie Y, Jiang Y, Lin L, Teng W, Cai C, Yao Y. Relation between iodine nutrition and thyroid diseases in Qinghai, China. Front Endocrinol (Lausanne). 2023;14:2. https://doi.org/10.3389/fendo.2023.1234482.
121. Gaertner R, Gasnier BCH, Dietrich JW, Krebs B, Angstwurm MWA. Selenium supplementation in patients with autoimmune thyroiditis decreases thyroid peroxidase antibodies concentrations. J Clin Endocrinol Metab. 2002;87:1687–91.
122. Toulis KA, Anastasilakis AD, Tzellos TG, Goulis DG, Kouvelas D. Selenium supplementation in the treatment of Hashimoto's thyroiditis: a systematic review and a meta-analysis. Thyroid. 2010;20:1163–73. https://doi.org/10.1089/thy.2009.0351.
123. Wichman J, Winther KH, Bonnema SJ, Hegedüs L. Selenium supplementation significantly reduces thyroid autoantibody levels in patients with chronic autoimmune thyroiditis: a systematic review and meta-analysis. Thyroid. 2016;26:1681–92. https://doi.org/10.1089/thy.2016.0256.
124. Duntas LH. The role of iodine and selenium in autoimmune thyroiditis. Horm Metab Res. 2015;47:721–6. https://doi.org/10.1055/s-0035-1559631.
125. Krysiak R, Szkróbka W, Okopień B. The effect of vitamin d and selenomethionine on thyroid antibody titers, hypothalamic-pituitary-thyroid axis activity and thyroid function tests in men with Hashimoto's thyroiditis: a pilot study. Pharmacol Rep. 2018;71:243–7. https://doi.org/10.1016/j.pharep.2018.10.012.
126. Huwiler VV, Maissen-Abgottspon S, Stanga Z, Mühlebach S, Trepp R, Bally L, Bano A. Selenium supplementation in patients with Hashimoto thyroiditis: a systematic review and meta-analysis of randomized clinical trials. Thyroid. 2024;34:295–313. https://doi.org/10.1089/thy.2023.0556.
127. Larsen C, Winther KH, Cramon PK, Rasmussen ÅK, Feldt-Rasmusssen U, Knudsen NJ, Bjorner JB, Schomburg L, Demircan K, Chillon TS, Gram J, Hansen SG, Brandt F, Nygaard B, Watt T, Hegedus L, Bonnema SJ. Selenium supplementation and placebo are equally effective in improving quality of life in patients with hypothyroidism. Eur Thyroid J. 2024;13:e230175. https://doi.org/10.1530/ETJ-23-0175.
128. Duntas LH. Reassessing selenium for the management of Hashimoto's thyroiditis: the selini shines bright for autoimmune thyroiditis patients. Thyroid. 2024;34:292–4. https://doi.org/10.1089/thy.2024.0078.
129. Duntas LH. The role of selenium in thyroid autoimmunity and cancer. Thyroid. 2006;16:455–60. https://doi.org/10.1089/thy.2006.16.455.
130. Larsen PR, Berry MJ. Nutritional and hormonal regulation of thyroid hormone deiodinases. Annu Rev Nutr. 1995;15:323–52. https://doi.org/10.1146/annurev.nu.15.070195.001543.
131. Wiersinga WM. Clinical relevance of environmental factors in the pathogenesis of autoimmune thyroid disease. Endocrinol Metab (Seoul). 2016;31:213–22. https://doi.org/10.3803/EnM.2016.31.2.213.
132. Hu S, Rayman MP. Multiple nutritional factors and the risk of Hashimoto's thyroiditis. Thyroid. 2017;27:597–610. https://doi.org/10.1089/thy.2016.0635.
133. Zhou Q, Xue S, Zhang L, Chen G. Trace elements and the thyroid. Front Endocrinol (Lausanne). 2022;13:904889. https://doi.org/10.3389/fendo.2022.904889.
134. Babić Leko M, Jureško I, Rozić I, Pleić N, Gunjača I, Zemunik T. Vitamin d and the thyroid: a critical review of the current evidence. Int J Mol Sci. 2023;24:3586. https://doi.org/10.3390/ijms24043586.
135. Kravchenko V, Zakharchenko T. Thyroid hormones and minerals in immunocorrection of disorders in autoimmune thyroid diseases. Front Endocrinol (Lausanne). 2023;14:1225494. https://doi.org/10.3389/fendo.2023.1225494.

136. Maric D, Baralic K, Javorac D, Mandic-Rajcevic S, Zarkovic M, Antonijevic B, Djukic-Cosic D, Bulat Z, Djordjevic AB. Nickel as a potential disruptor of thyroid function: benchmark modelling of human data. Front Endocrinol (Lausanne). 2023;14:1145153. https://doi.org/10.3389/fendo.2023.1145153.
137. Köhrle J. Selenium, iodine and iron-essential trace elements for thyroid hormone synthesis and metabolism. Int J Mol Sci. 2023;24:3393. https://doi.org/10.3390/ijms24043393.
138. Ye Y, Li Y, Ma Q, Li Y, Zeng H, Luo Y, Liang Y, Liu L, Liu L, Lin X, Yu G, Song C, Wan H, Shen J. Association of multiple blood metals with thyroid function in general adults: a cross-sectional study. Front Endocrinol (Lausanne). 2023;14:1134208. https://doi.org/10.3389/fendo.2023.1134208.
139. Schlienger JL, Grunenberger F, Vinzio S, Goichot B. Smoking and the thyroid. Ann Endocrinol (Paris). 2003;64:309–15.
140. Wu K, Zhou Y, Ke S, Huang J, Gao X, Li B, Lin X, Liu X, Liu X, Ma L, Wang L, Wu L, Wu L, Xie C, Xu J, Wang Y, Liu L. Lifestyle is associated with thyroid function in subclinical hypothyroidism: a cross-sectional study. BMC Endocr Disord. 2021;21:112. https://doi.org/10.1186/s12902-021-00772-z.
141. Ittermann T, Thamm M, Schipf S, John U, Rettig R, Völzke H. Relationship of smoking and/or passive exposure to tobacco smoke on the association between serum thyrotropin and body mass index in large groups of adolescents and children. Thyroid. 2013;23:262–8. https://doi.org/10.1089/thy.2012.0110.
142. Babić Leko MB, Gunjača I, Pleić N, Zemunik T. Environmental factors affecting thyroid-stimulating hormone and thyroid hormone levels. Int J Mol Sci. 2021;22:6521. https://doi.org/10.3390/ijms22126521.
143. Gore AC, Chappell VA, Fenton SE, Flaws JA, Nadal A, Prins GS, Toppari J, Zoeller RT. Edc-2: the endocrine society's second scientific statement on endocrine-disrupting chemicals. Endocr Rev. 2015;36:E1–E150. https://doi.org/10.1210/er.2015-1010.
144. Graceli JB, Dettogni RS, Merlo E, Niño O, Da Costa CS, Zanol JF, Morris EAR, Miranda-Alves L, Denicol AC. The impact of endocrine-disrupting chemical exposure in the mammalian hypothalamic-pituitary axis. Mol Cell Endocrinol. 2020;518:110997. https://doi.org/10.1016/j.mce.2020.110997.
145. Pitto L, Gorini F, Bianchi F, Guzzolino E. New insights into mechanisms of endocrine-disrupting chemicals in thyroid diseases: the epigenetic way. Int J Environ Res Public Health. 2020;17:7787. https://doi.org/10.3390/ijerph17217787.
146. Yuan N, Sun J, Zhao X, Li W. Relationship between bisphenol a and autoimmune thyroid disease in women of childbearing age. Front Endocrinol (Lausanne). 2024;15:1333915. https://doi.org/10.3389/fendo.2024.1333915.
147. Wysoczańska K, Tomaszewska-Zaremba D, Wójcik-Gładysz A. Metal nanoparticles—a real threat or harmless companions for the thyroid gland? A review. J Anim Feed Sci. 2024; https://doi.org/10.22358/jafs/193929/2024.

Chapter 12
Special Considerations in the Treatment of Hypothyroidism

Rudolf Hoermann and Johannes W. Dietrich

12.1 The Athyreotic Patient

The total loss of functional thyroid tissue is particularly challenging for a patient. It leaves the patient in a state of *athyroidism* and entirely dependent on external hormone supply. It also breaks the homeostatic regulation of the hypothalamic–pituitary–thyroid axis, especially with respect to thyroid-stimulating hormone (TSH) signalling, FT3 stability, and FT3 homeostasis [1, 2]. The pathophysiology of this condition has been explored and explained in preceding chapters on relational stability and hypothalamic–pituitary–thyroid regulation. Main *causes* for an irreversible loss of thyroid function are a long history of thyroid autoimmune disease with progressive destruction of thyroid tissue and ablative treatments such as total thyroidectomy and radioiodine administration for malignant or less frequently benign thyroid disease.

R. Hoermann (✉)
Yandina, QLD, Australia

Department of General Internal Medicine, Gastroenterology and Endocrinology, [Retired] Klinikum Lüdenscheid, Lüdenscheid, Germany
e-mail: rudolf.hoermann@gmail.com

J. W. Dietrich
Diabetes, Endocrinology and Metabolism Section, Department of Medicine, St. Josef-Hospital, Ruhr University Hospitals, Bochum, Germany

Centre for Diabetes Technology (ZDT), Catholic Hospitals Bochum, Bochum, Germany

Centre for Rare Endocrine Diseases (ZSEK), Ruhr Center for Rare Diseases (CeSER), Ruhr University of Bochum and Witten/Herdecke University, Bochum, Germany

Centre for Thyroid Medicine (ZSM), Ruhr University of Bochum, Bochum, Germany
e-mail: johannes.dietrich@ruhr-uni-bochum.de

R. Hoermann, J. W. Dietrich (eds.), *Hypothyroidism*,
https://doi.org/10.1007/978-981-96-3682-2_12

In patients with *thyroid carcinoma*, the treatment concept for differentiated thyroid cancers (DTCs) consists of surgery, post-operative adjuvant radioactive iodine treatment and long-term hormonal replacement after ablative treatment [3–12]. Depending on the stage of their cancer, many thyroid carcinoma patients require total thyroidectomy resulting in severe primary hypothyroidism and rendering them dependent on external thyroid hormone supply. Calcitonin replacement is currently not recommended after total thyroidectomy, which results in a loss of C cells. Post-operative hypoparathyroidism is a surgical complication with transient or permanent hypocalcaemia (1–5%). It is treated with calcium and vitamin D supplementation.

In patients undergoing thyroidectomy due to benign thyroid disease, the outcome is more variable, depending on the amount of residual thyroid tissue after surgery [13]. Patients with *hemithyroidectomy* may present with a moderately raised TSH levels after the surgery but may be able to avoid LT4 substitution. Owing to the increased TSH stimulation, the remaining thyroid tissue may slowly grow, as evidenced by a fall in the TSH concentrations over time [14–16]. Higher pre-operative TSH levels, older age, female sex, presence of autoimmune thyroiditis, TPO Ab and Tg Ab, and right-sided hemithyroidectomy were associated with higher risk of post-operative hypothyroidism [17].

Patients taking *drugs interfering with thyroid function* may suffer from more or less severe transient or permanent forms of hypothyroidism [18, 19]. The condition is not always reversible after the cessation of the drug. Particularly hypothyroidism in association with checkpoint inhibitors for oncological indications may frequently develop autoimmune thyroid disease and require permanent substitution with thyroid hormones.

12.1.1 Treatment Problems in Athyreotic Patients

Due to several impediments and disrupted mechanisms of thyroid homeostasis, the treatment of *athyreotic patients* is more challenging. The probability of incomplete symptom relief on standard LT4 treatment increases in these patients.

The situation has worsened for thyroid cancer patients after guidelines have relaxed their former position on the requirement of maintaining TSH-suppressive treatment targets in these patients to suppress any potential TSH-induced regrowth of differentiated thyroid tumour cells and risk of relapse of the cancer [4, 20–22]. TSH-suppressive LT4 treatment is now recommended only for more advanced thyroid cancers. However, the optimum TSH level for patients with low-risk differentiated papillary thyroid carcinoma is still a matter of debate [23, 24]. Blocking the human TSH receptor, on the other hand, has been experimentally shown to inhibit the proliferation of thyroid tumour cells and metastasis in vitro and in vivo [25]. Thyroid malignancies other than differentiated thyroid cancer (DTC) do not respond to the TSH stimulus. Parallel with these policy changes, the *spectrum of symptoms* experienced by athyreotic patients on LT4 treatment has changed [21]. While the prevalence of hyperthyroid symptoms has declined, residual hypothyroid complaints are now much more frequently reported by patients.

Athyreotic patients display substantial variations in their *T3 conversion efficiency* on LT4 treatment [26]. More than 20% of these patients, despite achieving normal TSH levels, could not maintain their FT3 concentrations in the reference range [27–29]. Athyreotic patients are particularly susceptible to hormonal imbalance and regulatory disturbances due to their loss of a functioning thyroid gland [1, 13, 30]. One of the consequences of thyroidectomy is that it *breaks FT3 homeostasis* [2]. In particular, the loss of the intra-thyroidal TSH-T3 shunt (TSH feed-forward) and inability to increase compensatory T3 secretion by the thyroid gland shifts the balance between TSH, FT4, and FT3 levels, compared to that prior to surgery [31] (Chap. 2). The personal working points are altered in the same patient from health to disease, i.e. before and after thyroidectomy [28, 30]. The equilibria in individuals appropriate for their healthy state do not remain unaltered and cannot therefore act as equivalent targets for their diseased state [32]. This explains why *their former TSH level is no longer indicative of the euthyroid state*, and these patients may continue to suffer from residual symptoms [13]. Consequently, athyreotic patients frequently develop a *low-FT3 state under LT4 substitution* even after their TSH levels have been normalised with LT4 replacement [27–29, 33–35].

Prioritising apparent TSH "normalisation" as a treatment goal over restoring FT3 homeostasis frequently denies these patients adequate FT3 normalisation, which does not help their symptoms. Rather the interpretation of a given TSH value should be conditional, as appropriate to the clinical situation and the resulting FT4 and FT3 levels [1, 2, 36].

To raise the FT3 level after thyroidectomy to the same level it had been prior to thyroidectomy, many patients on LT4 may need a suppressed TSH to achieve this goal [28, 30]. This per se does not mean thyrotoxicosis to them *if their balance point has shifted* in the absence of TSH feed-forward onto FT3 and their FT3 concentration remains in range [37]. Often it is already sufficient to raise the level of FT3 from below reference or close to its lower limit to midrange [38]. However, given the individualised dosing requirements, narrow therapeutic range of thyroid hormones and potential adverse effects associated with thyrotoxicosis *overdosing* has to be avoided by monitoring FT3 concentrations together with FT4 and TSH [39].

In some patients, escalation of the LT4 dose may not have the desired effect on FT3 concentrations, rather *paradoxically* lowering their FT3 levels while further increasing their FT4 serum concentrations [26]. This leads to a progressive *TSH-FT3 disjoint* and an *abnormal FT3 to FT4 ratio*. A possible explanation for the phenomenon may be monodeiodination of FT4 at the outer ring producing rT3 instead of FT3. The latter may, in turn, block the activity of deiodinase type 2 and some actions of T3. Genetic factors may play an additional role [40–42]. The FT3 to FT4 ratio or calculated step-up deiodinase activity (SPINA-GD) is therefore an important additional marker to uncover these issues [43] (Sect. 10.3). These patients are candidates for additional *T3 supplementation* and alternative drugs to remedy the situation.

12.2 Pregnant Patients

Numerous metabolic and energetic requirements increase during pregnancy [44–46]. The *demand for thyroid hormones increases* by as much as 50% during that period [47]. Physiologically, the required increase in the functional thyroid capacity is associated with *glandular hypertrophy* and an enlarged thyroid volume of approx. 10–15%. This fact has not gone unnoticed by ancient civilisations. Egyptian women for instance wearing a tight reed necklace used its rupture as a "pregnancy test".

The placenta of the foetus is given additional control over the thyroid hormone synthesis and secretion of the mother's thyroid, with the pregnancy hormone human chorionic gonadotropin (hCG) and its variant forms acting as TSH receptor agonists similar to the actions of pituitary TSH [48–50]. The *dual thyroid regulation by TSH and hCG* in pregnancy is shown in Fig. 12.1. As a result of thyroidal stimulation by placental hCG, TSH concentrations show a physiological decline in early pregnancy between the 8th and 14th week of gestation, returning back to their original level only in the second and third trimester [51]. The uncontrolled placental stimulation of the thyroid may result in complete suppression of TSH and in 1–2% of women in a special form of transient pregnancy-related hyperthyroidism [52–57]. HCG-induced *gestational hyperthyroidism* is associated with the syndrome of *hyperemesis gravidarum*. This type of hyperthyroidism is not to be confused with an oestrogen-induced increase in TBG concentrations and *euthyroid*

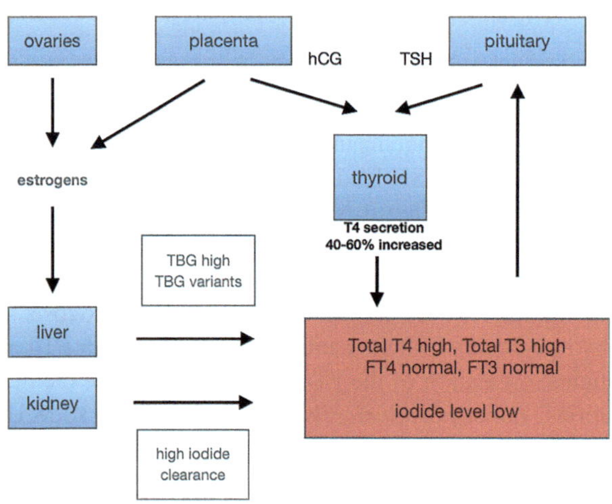

Fig. 12.1 Physiological thyroid regulation in pregnancy
In early pregnancy, the thyroid is stimulated by two hormones, pituitary TSH and placental hCG to increase its output of thyroid hormones. Binding proteins (TBGs) are increased due to induction in the liver by oestrogens, raising circulating total T4 and total T3 concentrations, termed hyperthyroxinaemia, and not to be confused with the elevation of FT4, FT3 concentrations and the disease hyperthyroidism. Iodine is frequently deficient due to high demand and more rapid clearance

hyperthyroxinemia, resulting in an increase in circulating total T4 and total T3 concentrations, but not FT4 and FT3.

Iodide concentrations decline substantially in the bloodstream of the mother due to increased renal clearance and additional demands of the foetus. This may lead to a *relative hypothyroxinaemia* during pregnancy [51, 58]. Routine *iodine supplements* taken as a prophylactic measure and provision of adequate iodine supply are therefore important to avoid potential hypothyroidism in pregnancy. This *prophylaxis* should even be maintained in patients with thyroid autoimmune disease, with a daily dose of 100–150 μg/day of iodine.

The placenta is a *barrier* between the maternal and foetal blood circulation. TSH and maternal thyroid hormones show little transfer across the placenta under normal conditions. Congenital foetal hypothyroidism may be an exception where sufficient thyroid hormone concentrations are achieved in the foetal blood to avoid severe signs of foetal hypothyroidism. In contrast, iodine, TRH, TSH receptor antibodies, and anti-thyroid drugs (thiamazole more so than propylthiouracil) readily pass the placenta.

12.2.1 Hypothyroidism in Pregnancy

Latent or pre-existing hypothyroidism will deteriorate in pregnancy due to *increased physiological thyroid hormone requirements* during that period. This may require thyroid hormone substitution to be commenced or LT4 dosage taken prior to the pregnancy to be increased by, on average, 50 μg/day. Dose adjustments should be monitored and individualised [44–46, 59–64]. It is particularly important that the mother maintains a euthyroid function during pregnancy since maternal hypothyroidism has been associated with long-term cognitive deficits of children [65]. It is recommended that when a hypothyroid patient plans a pregnancy, TSH, being the most sensitive indicator, is measured prior to conception and the substitution dosage adjusted accordingly.

12.2.2 Post-Partum Thyroiditis

A specific form of thyroiditis may be experienced by up to 10% of mothers' post-partum [66]. The aetiology of the disease is a cytotoxic autoimmune reaction, which, unlike autoimmune thyroiditis, is self-limiting after 2–3 months in approximately 95% of all patients. The clinical manifestation is often mild and unapparent. Notably the disease may begin with a short-lived thyrotoxic phase, to be symptomatically treated with the administration of beta-blockers. Anti-thyroid drugs are not effective. The second hypothyroid phase is treated by substitution of thyroid hormones as needed. The third phase of recovery usually allows for the substitution to be discontinued. Thyroid peroxidase antibodies (TPO Ab) may be found to be slightly elevated in the disease.

Post-partum thyroiditis is suspected by the typical time of its occurrence. It must be differentiated from pre-existing autoimmune thyroiditis (higher TPO Ab levels than typically found in post-partum thyroiditis) and Graves' disease (increased iodine uptake, as opposed to the low uptake in post-partum thyroiditis even in the hyperthyroid phase). de Quervain's thyroiditis, unlike post-partum thyroiditis, is much more painful and shows strongly elevated inflammatory markers such as C-reactive protein (CRP). Post-partum thyroiditis may occasionally trigger, via increased antigen presentation, secondary Graves' disease, or T-cell-mediated autoimmune thyroiditis.

12.2.3 Secondary Hypothyroidism

Secondary hypothyroidism arises from the event of peripartal pituitary deficiency, also known as *Sheehan syndrome*, or due to hypophysitis [67]. An indicative feature of suspicion of the disease is the inability of the mother to breastfeed her baby (due to prolactin deficiency). FT4 concentration is found to be low in these patients, while TSH levels are low or normal. Other pituitary hormones are also affected in most patients. LT4 is substituted only after the restoration of cortisol sufficiency with the administration of hydrocortisone.

12.2.4 Hypothyroidism Post-Thyroidectomy

Thyroid surgery is rarely performed in pregnant women, unless deemed urgent for instance due to an aggressive thyroid malignancy [68].

12.2.5 Laboratory Diagnostics in Pregnancy

Pregnancy-specific reference ranges for TSH and thyroid hormones are available and to be used according to the week of gestation [69–76]. TSH shows a characteristic mirror image to hCG, with a rise of the latter and fall of the former in early pregnancy [51].

12.3 Paediatric Patients

12.3.1 Hypothyroidism Due to Premature Birth

The *premature birth* of the baby may be associated with a form of hypothyroidism due to both developmental retardation and non-thyroidal illness syndrome (TACITUS), which is transient and will improve without intervention [77].

12.3.2 Congenital Hypothyroidism

Congenital hypothyroidism affects 1:2000–1:4000 newborns, girls and boys in a ratio of 2 to 1 [78–81]. The hidden disease is uncovered with screening programmes for newborns that have long been established in many countries [79, 82]. Comorbidity has also to be considered [83]. A missed diagnosis and lack of adequate treatment causes severe long-term neurological, motor developmental, and mental retardation. Adverse outcomes can be prevented by early diagnosis and treatment. At birth, symptoms are mostly absent or subtle, making diagnosis difficult and reliant on *screening*.

A cut-off level of 10 mIU/l TSH is recommended for screening to be followed by additional confirmatory testing, showing TSH levels greater than 15 mIU/L and total or free T4 concentrations with normal or low values. Resistance to thyroid hormone has to be considered in the differential diagnosis [84].

Congenital hypothyroidism can be permanent or transient. Its *aetiology* is classified as primary, secondary, or tertiary [85–87]. The permanent disease requires both early and lifelong treatment, while transient forms recover within months or years.

The aetiology of permanent congenital hypothyroidism comprises

- Thyroid dysgenesis (TD) corresponding to 85% of cases
- Dyshormonogenesis (DH) representing 10–15% of cases [88]
- Secondary pituitary and tertiary hypothalamic dysfunctions, which are rare and commonly associated with other pituitary deficiencies

Approximately 85% of cases are sporadic, while 15% are hereditary [78].

Both aetiology and clinical phenotype determine the severity of disease and response to treatment [89, 90]. Children may need close monitoring and substitution with higher doses, especially in early life to achieve adequate neurological development [91–95]. Inadequate hormone levels lead to specific brain dysfunctions in regions such as the posterior parietal, inferior temporal lobes, caudate nucleus, and hippocampus, responsible for, respectively, spatial location, object identification, attention, and memory. Some forms of congenital hypothyroidism are accompanied by *hearing loss* [96]. Occasionally, hypothyroidism may manifest with *precocious puberty* (Van Wyk–Grumbach syndrome) [97].

Specific laboratory reference ranges apply to neonates and paediatric populations [90, 94, 98–102].

In children, clinical monitoring of any form of hypothyroidism should address *developmental aspects* and signs of *growth retardation* in addition to typical hypothyroid signs and symptoms. Dose recommendation for the treatment of congenital hypothyroidism with levothyroxine are age-dependent, to be additionally adjusted on an individual basis.

12.4 Older patients

The diagnosis and treatment of hypothyroidism in elderly patients face *several challenges* [18, 103–115].

1. The *prevalence* of hypothyroidism, particularly due to autoimmune thyroid disease increases with age.
2. The *responsiveness* of the hypothalamic–pituitary–thyroid axis in the regulation of both thyroid hormones and TSH is diminished and range compressed.
3. Hypothyroid *symptoms* in older patients are often subtle and overlap with signs of the ageing process.
4. *Requirements* for thyroid hormone substitution are reduced in the older population.
5. Non-thyroidal *comorbidity* may interfere with the diagnostic process, for instance in patients with a low-T3 syndrome due to non-thyroidal illness.
6. Use of *non-thyroidal medication* and drug-related interferences with thyroid function or thyroid function testing are more prevalent than in a younger population.

Laboratory-based diagnostics should include some guidance from attempts to establish *age-related reference ranges* [95, 116–120].

12.4.1 Treatment of Hypothyroidism in the Elderly

1. The treatment of the elderly patients is generally similar to the standard treatment in adults with some notable exceptions.
2. There are no contraindications to a required treatment of overt hypothyroidism.
3. Dose requirements for levothyroxine may *decrease* by as much as 30% to achieve the same biochemical targets as in younger patients.
4. The target dose may need to be reached *more gradually* due to the possibly longer pre-existence of the hypothyroid condition and potential cardiac comorbidity reducing the tolerance of thyroid hormones.

5. Development of new *cardiac symptomatology*, such as angina pectoris or its worsening, should trigger both an adjustment of the levothyroxine dose and a thorough cardiological examination and potential intervention.

References

1. Hoermann R, Midgley JEM, Larisch R, Dietrich JW. Relational stability in the expression of normality, variation, and control of thyroid function. Front Endocrinol (Lausanne). 2016;7:142. https://doi.org/10.3389/fendo.2016.00142.
2. Hoermann R, Pekker MJ, Midgley JEM, Dietrich JW. The role of supporting and disruptive mechanisms of FT3 homeostasis in regulating the hypothalamic-pituitary-thyroid axis. Ther Adv Endocrinol Metab. 2023;14:20420188231158163. https://doi.org/10.1177/20420188231158163.
3. Van Nostrand D, Wartofsky L. Radioiodine in the treatment of thyroid cancer. Endocrinol Metab Clin N Am. 2007;36:807–22.
4. Haugen BR, Alexander EK, Bible KC, Doherty GM, Mandel SJ, Nikiforov YE, Pacini F, Randolph GW, Sawka AM, Schlumberger M, Schuff KG, Sherman SI, Sosa JA, Steward DL, Tuttle RM, Wartofsky L. 2015 American Thyroid Association management guidelines for adult patients with thyroid nodules and differentiated thyroid cancer: The American Thyroid Association guidelines task force on thyroid nodules and differentiated thyroid cancer. Thyroid. 2016;26:1–133. https://doi.org/10.1089/thy.2015.0020.
5. Cabanillas ME, Mcfadden DG, Durante C. Thyroid cancer. Lancet. 2016;388:2783–95.
6. Haymart MR, Esfandiari NH, Stang MT, Sosa JA. Controversies in the management of low-risk differentiated thyroid cancer. Endocr Rev. 2017;38:351–78. https://doi.org/10.1210/er.2017-00067.
7. Schmidbauer B, Menhart K, Hellwig D, Grosse J. Differentiated thyroid cancer—treatment: State of the art. Int J Mol Sci. 2017;18:1292.
8. Wang TS, Sosa JA. Thyroid surgery for differentiated thyroid cancer—recent advances and future directions. Nat Rev Endocrinol. 2018;14:670–83. https://doi.org/10.1038/s41574-018-0080-7.
9. Araque KA, Gubbi S, Klubo-Gwiezdzinska J. Updates on the management of thyroid cancer. Horm Metab Res. 2020;52:562–77.
10. Bednarczuk T. Levothyroxine and cancer. In: 70 years of levothyroxine. Cham: Springer; 2021. p. 109–20.
11. Schlumberger M, Leboulleux S. Current practice in patients with differentiated thyroid cancer. Nat Rev Endocrinol. 2021;17:176–88. https://doi.org/10.1038/s41574-020-00448-z.
12. Chou R, Dana T, Haymart M, Leung AM, Tufano RP, Sosa JA, Ringel MD. Active surveillance versus thyroid surgery for differentiated thyroid cancer: a systematic review. Thyroid. 2022;32:351–67.
13. Ito M, Miyauchi A, Kang S, Hisakado M, Yoshioka W, Ide A, Kudo T, Nishihara E, Kihara M, Ito Y, Kobayashi K, Miya A, Fukata S, Nakamura H, Amino N. Effect of the presence of remnant thyroid tissue on the serum thyroid hormone balance in thyroidectomized patients. Eur J Endocrinol. 2015;173:333–40. https://doi.org/10.1530/EJE-15-0138.
14. Ahn D, Sohn JH, Jeon JH. Hypothyroidism following hemithyroidectomy: incidence, risk factors, and clinical characteristics. J Clin Endocrinol Metab. 2016;101:1429–36. https://doi.org/10.1210/jc.2015-3997.
15. Park S, Jeon MJ, Song E, Oh H-S, Kim M, Kwon H, Kim TY, Hong SJ, Shong YK, Kim WB, Sung T-Y, Kim WG. Clinical features of early and late postoperative hypothyroidism after lobectomy. J Clin Endocrinol Metab. 2017;102:1317–24. https://doi.org/10.1210/jc.2016-3597.

16. Kostev K, Winiarski M, Schüller L, Sesterhenn AM, Jacob L. Frequency of thyroid-stimulating hormone monitoring in patients after thyroidectomy: a retrospective study in primary care practices in Germany. Exp Clin Endocrinol Diabetes. 2018;126:640–4. https://doi.org/10.1055/s-0044-100038.
17. Cooper D, Kaur R, Ayeni FE, Eslick GD, Edirimanne S. Hypothyroidism after hemithyroidectomy: a systematic review and meta-analysis. Thyroid Res. 2024;17:18. https://doi.org/10.1186/s13044-024-00200-z.
18. Benvenga S. L-T4 therapy in the presence of pharmacological interferents. Front Endocrinol (Lausanne). 2020;11:607446. https://doi.org/10.3389/fendo.2020.607446.
19. Tsai K, Ma H, Liang TZ, Xing Y, Chung S, Dorff T, Bell D, Lechner MG. The combined effect of immune checkpoint inhibitors and tyrosine kinase inhibitors on thyroid function. Thyroid. 2024;34:158–66. https://doi.org/10.1089/thy.2023.0542.
20. Durante C, Costante G, Filetti S. Differentiated thyroid carcinoma: defining new paradigms for postoperative management. Endocr Relat Cancer. 2013;20:R141–54. https://doi.org/10.1530/ERC-13-0066.
21. Midgley JEM, Toft AD, Larisch R, Dietrich JW, Hoermann R. Time for a reassessment of the treatment of hypothyroidism. BMC Endocr Disord. 2019;19:37. https://doi.org/10.1186/s12902-019-0365-4.
22. Monzani ML, Piccinini F, Boselli G, Corleto R, Margiotta G, Peeters RP, Simoni M, Brigante G. Changes in quality of life after thyroidectomy in subjects with thyroid cancer in relation to the dose of levothyroxine. J Endocrinol Investig. 2023;46:319–26. https://doi.org/10.1007/s40618-022-01903-6.
23. Miyauchi A. Response to Xiang and Zhang re:"active surveillance outcomes of patients with low-risk papillary thyroid microcarcinoma according to levothyroxine treatment status". Thyroid. 2024;38:673–8. https://doi.org/10.1089/thy.2023.0697.
24. Xiang J, Zhang H. Re: "active surveillance outcomes of patients with low-risk papillary thyroid microcarcinoma according to levothyroxine treatment status" by Yamamoto et al. Thyroid. 2024;34:399–400. https://doi.org/10.1089/thy.2023.0605.
25. Sarkar R, Bolel P, Kapoor A, Eliseeva E, Dulcey AE, Templin JS, Wang AQ, Xu X, Southall N, Klubo-Gwiezdzinska J, Neumann S, Marugan JJ, Gershengorn MC. An orally efficacious thyrotropin receptor ligand inhibits growth and metastatic activity of thyroid cancers. J Clin Endocrinol Metab. 2024;109:2306–16. https://doi.org/10.1210/clinem/dgae114.
26. Midgley JEM, Larisch R, Dietrich JW, Hoermann R. Variation in the biochemical response to L-thyroxine therapy and relationship with peripheral thyroid hormone conversion efficiency. Endocr Connect. 2015;4:196–205. https://doi.org/10.1530/EC-15-0056.
27. Gullo D, Latina A, Frasca F, Le Moli R, Pellegriti G, Vigneri R. Levothyroxine monotherapy cannot guarantee euthyroidism in all athyreotic patients. PLoS One. 2011;6:e22552. https://doi.org/10.1371/journal.pone.0022552.
28. Ito M, Miyauchi A, Morita S, Kudo T, Nishihara E, Kihara M, Takamura Y, Ito Y, Kobayashi K, Miya A, Kubota S, Amino N. TSH-suppressive doses of levothyroxine are required to achieve preoperative native serum triiodothyronine levels in patients who have undergone total thyroidectomy. Eur J Endocrinol. 2012;167:373–8. https://doi.org/10.1530/EJE-11-1029.
29. Hoermann R, Midgley JEM, Larisch R, Dietrich JW. Is pituitary TSH an adequate measure of thyroid hormone-controlled homoeostasis during thyroxine treatment. Eur J Endocrinol. 2013;168:271–80. https://doi.org/10.1530/EJE-12-0819.
30. Ito M, Miyauchi A, Hisakado M, Yoshioka W, Ide A, Kudo T, Nishihara E, Kihara M, Ito Y, Kobayashi K, Miya A, Fukata S, Nishikawa M, Nakamura H, Amino N. Biochemical markers reflecting thyroid function in athyreotic patients on levothyroxine monotherapy. Thyroid. 2017;27:484–90. https://doi.org/10.1089/thy.2016.0426.
31. Hoermann R, Pekker MJ, Midgley JEM, Larisch R, Dietrich JW. Triiodothyronine secretion in early thyroid failure: the adaptive response of central feedforward control. Eur J Clin Investig. 2020;50:e13192. https://doi.org/10.1111/eci.13192.

32. Hoermann R, Midgley JEM, Larisch R, Dietrich JW. Recent advances in thyroid hormone regulation: toward a new paradigm for optimal diagnosis and treatment. Front Endocrinol (Lausanne). 2017;8:364. https://doi.org/10.3389/fendo.2017.00364.
33. Peterson SJ, Mcaninch EA, Bianco AC. Is a normal TSH synonymous with "euthyroidism" in levothyroxine monotherapy. J Clin Endocrinol Metab. 2016;101:4964–73. https://doi.org/10.1210/jc.2016-2660.
34. Casula S, Ettleson MD, Bianco AC. Are we restoring thyroid hormone signaling in levothyroxine-treated patients with residual symptoms of hypothyroidism? Endocr Pract. 2023;29:581–8. https://doi.org/10.1016/j.eprac.2023.04.003.
35. Penna GC, Bensenor IM, Bianco AC, Ettleson MD. Thyroid hormone homeostasis in levothyroxine-treated patients: findings from Elsa-Brasil. J Clin Endocrinol Metab. 2024:dgae139. https://doi.org/10.1210/clinem/dgae139/7632160.
36. Hoermann R, Midgley JEM, Larisch R, Dietrich JW. Advances in applied homeostatic modelling of the relationship between thyrotropin and free thyroxine. PLoS One. 2017;12:e0187232. https://doi.org/10.1371/journal.pone.0187232.
37. Hoermann R, Midgley JEM, Larisch R, Dietrich JW. Heterogenous biochemical expression of hormone activity in subclinical/overt hyperthyroidism and exogenous thyrotoxicosis. J Clin Transl Endocrinol. 2020;19:100219. https://doi.org/10.1016/j.jcte.2020.100219.
38. Hoermann R, Midgley JEM, Larisch R, Dietrich JW. Functional and symptomatic individuality in the response to levothyroxine treatment. Front Endocrinol (Lausanne). 2019;10:664. https://doi.org/10.3389/fendo.2019.00664.
39. Hoermann R, Midgley JEM, Larisch R, Dietrich JW. Individualised requirements for optimum treatment of hypothyroidism: complex needs, limited options. Drugs Context. 2019;8:212597. https://doi.org/10.7573/dic.212597.
40. Kim BW, Bianco AC. For some, L-thyroxine replacement might not be enough: a genetic rationale. J Clin Endocrinol Metab. 2009;94:1521–3. https://doi.org/10.1210/jc.2009-0410.
41. Medici M, Visser WE, Visser TJ, Peeters RP. Genetic determination of the hypothalamic-pituitary-thyroid axis: where do we stand? Endocr Rev. 2015;36:214–44. https://doi.org/10.1210/er.2014-1081.
42. Lacámara N, Lecumberri B, Barquiel B, Escribano A, González-Casado I, Álvarez-Escolá C, Aleixandre-Blanquer F, Morales F, Alfayate R, Bernal-Soriano MC, Miralles R, Yildirim Simsir I, Özgen AG, Bernal J, Berbel P, Moreno JC. Identification of resistance to exogenous thyroxine in humans. Thyroid. 2020;30:1732–44. https://doi.org/10.1089/thy.2019.0825.
43. Dietrich JW, Landgrafe-Mende G, Wiora E, Chatzitomaris A, Klein HH, Midgley JEM, Hoermann R. Calculated parameters of thyroid homeostasis: emerging tools for differential diagnosis and clinical research. Front Endocrinol (Lausanne). 2016;7:57. https://doi.org/10.3389/fendo.2016.00057.
44. Alexander EK, Pearce EN, Brent GA, Brown RS, Chen H, Dosiou C, Grobman WA, Laurberg P, Lazarus JH, Mandel SJ, Peeters RP, Sullivan S. 2017 guidelines of the American Thyroid Association for the diagnosis and management of thyroid disease during pregnancy and the postpartum. Thyroid. 2017;27:315–89. https://doi.org/10.1089/thy.2016.0457.
45. Muller I, Taylor PN, Lazarus JH. Thyroid function in pregnancy. Ann Thyroid. 2018;3:27. https://doi.org/10.21037/aot.2018.10.05.
46. Ahn HY, Yi KH. Diagnosis and management of thyroid disease during pregnancy and postpartum: 2023 revised Korean thyroid association guidelines. Endocrinol Metab (Seoul). 2023;38:289–94. https://doi.org/10.3803/EnM.2023.1696.
47. Fantz CR, Dagogo-Jack S, Ladenson JH, Gronowski AM. Thyroid function during pregnancy. Clin Chem. 1999;45:2250–8.
48. Mann K, Hoermann R. Thyroid stimulation by placental factors. J Endocrinol Investig. 1993;16:378–84. https://doi.org/10.1007/BF03348862.
49. Hoermann R, Poertl S, Liss I, Amir SM, Mann K. Variation in the thyrotropic activity of human chorionic gonadotropin in Chinese hamster ovary cells arises from differential

expression of the human thyrotropin receptor and microheterogeneity of the hormone. J Clin Endocrinol Metab. 1995;80:1605–10. https://doi.org/10.1210/jcem.80.5.7745007.

50. Casarini L, Santi D, Brigante G, Simoni M. Two hormones for one receptor: evolution, biochemistry, actions, and pathophysiology of LH and hCG. Endocr Rev. 2018;39:549–92. https://doi.org/10.1210/er.2018-00065.
51. Glinoer D, De Nayer P, Bourdoux P, Lemone M, Robyn C, Van Steirteghem A, Kinthaert J, Lejeune B. Regulation of maternal thyroid during pregnancy. J Clin Endocrinol Metab. 1990;71:276–87.
52. Kato K, Mostafa MH, Mann K, Schindler AE, Hoermann R. The human chorionic gonadotropin molecule from patients with trophoblastic diseases has a high thyrotropic activity but is less active in the ovary. Gynecol Endocrinol. 2004;18:269–77. https://doi.org/10.1080/09513590410001667247.
53. Walkington L, Webster J, Hancock BW, Everard J, Coleman RE. Hyperthyroidism and human chorionic gonadotrophin production in gestational trophoblastic disease. Br J Cancer. 2011;104:1665–9. https://doi.org/10.1038/bjc.2011.139.
54. Labadzhyan A, Brent GA, Hershman JM, Leung AM. Thyrotoxicosis of pregnancy. J Clin Transl Endocrinol. 2014;1:140–4. https://doi.org/10.1016/j.jcte.2014.07.008.
55. Korevaar TIM, De Rijke YB, Chaker L, Medici M, Jaddoe VWV, Steegers EAP, Visser TJ, Peeters RP. Stimulation of thyroid function by human chorionic gonadotropin during pregnancy: a risk factor for thyroid disease and a mechanism for known risk factors. Thyroid. 2017;27:440–50. https://doi.org/10.1089/thy.2016.0527.
56. Uldall Torp NM, Liew Z, Carlé A, Karmisholt J, Pedersen IB, Andersen S, Andersen SL. Hyperthyroidism in Danish pregnant women during a 20-year period. J Clin Endocrinol Metab. 2023;109:e370–8. https://doi.org/10.1210/clinem/dgad410.
57. Cohen-Sela E, Brener A, Raviv O, Yackobovitch-Gavan M, Almashanu S, Marom R, Anteby M, Hiersch L, Lebenthal Y. Outcomes in maternal Graves' disease: a population-based mother-infant dyad cohort study. Thyroid. 2024;34:123–33. https://doi.org/10.1089/thy.2023.0291.
58. Pop VJ, Hulsbosch LP, Boekhorst MGBM, Broeren MAC, Krabbe JG, Wiersinga WM. Hypothyroid symptoms throughout pregnancy are predominantly associated with thyroxine and not with thyrotropin concentrations. Thyroid. 2022;32:1249–58. https://doi.org/10.1089/thy.2022.0244.
59. Haddow JE, Palomaki GE, Allan WC, Williams JR, Knight GJ, Gagnon J, O'heir CE, Mitchell ML, Hermos RJ, Waisbren SE, Faix JD, Klein RZ. Maternal thyroid deficiency during pregnancy and subsequent neuropsychological development of the child. N Engl J Med. 1999;341:549–55.
60. Glinoer D. Potential consequences of maternal hypothyroidism on the offspring: evidence and implications. Horm Res. 2001;55:109–14.
61. Azizi F, Amouzegar A. Management of hyperthyroidism during pregnancy and lactation. Eur J Endocrinol. 2011;164:871–6. https://doi.org/10.1530/EJE-10-1030.
62. Stagnaro-Green A, Pearce E. Thyroid disorders in pregnancy. Nat Rev Endocrinol. 2012;8:650–8. https://doi.org/10.1038/nrendo.2012.171.
63. Korevaar TI, Chaker L, Medici M, De Rijke YB, Jaddoe VW, Steegers EA, Tiemeier H, Visser TJ, Peeters RP. Maternal total T4 during the first half of pregnancy: physiologic aspects and the risk of adverse outcomes in comparison with free T4. Clin Endocrinol. 2016;85:757–63. https://doi.org/10.1111/cen.13106.
64. Rotondi M, Chiovato L, Pacini F, Bartalena L, Vitti P. Management of subclinical hypothyroidism in pregnancy: a comment from the Italian society of endocrinology and the Italian thyroid association to the 2017 American Thyroid Association guidelines—"the Italian way". Thyroid. 2018;28:551–5. https://doi.org/10.1089/thy.2017.0424.
65. Päkkilä F, Männistö T, Surcel H-M, Ruokonen A, Bloigu A, Pouta A, Hartikainen A-L, Vääräsmäki M, Järvelin M-R, Suvanto E. Maternal thyroid dysfunction during pregnancy

and thyroid function of her child in adolescence. J Clin Endocrinol Metab. 2013;98:965–72. https://doi.org/10.1210/jc.2012-2028.
66. Stagnaro-Green A. Clinical review 152: postpartum thyroiditis. J Clin Endocrinol Metab. 2002;87:4042–7. https://doi.org/10.1210/jc.2002-020524.
67. Shivaprasad C. Sheehan's syndrome: newer advances. Indian J Endocrinol Metab. 2011;15(Suppl 3):S203–7. https://doi.org/10.4103/2230-8210.84869.
68. Kuy S, Roman SA, Desai R, Sosa JA. Outcomes following thyroid and parathyroid surgery in pregnant women. Arch Surg. 2009;144:399–406; discussion 406. https://doi.org/10.1001/archsurg.2009.48.
69. Gilbert RM, Hadlow NC, Walsh JP, Fletcher SJ, Brown SJ, Stuckey BG, Lim EM. Assessment of thyroid function during pregnancy: first-trimester (weeks 9-13) reference intervals derived from western Australian women. Med J Aust. 2008;189:250–3. https://doi.org/10.5694/j.1326-5377.2008.tb02015.x.
70. Kennedy RL, Malabu UH, Porter D. Assessment of thyroid function during pregnancy: first-trimester (weeks 9-13) reference intervals derived from western Australian women. Comment Med J Aust. 2009;190:219–20. https://doi.org/10.5694/j.1326-5377.2009.tb02357.x.
71. Bocos-Terraz JP, Izquierdo-Álvarez S, Bancalero-Flores JL, Álvarez-Lahuerta R, Aznar-Sauca A, Real-López E, Ibáñez-Marco R, Bocanegra-García V, Rivera-Sánchez G. Thyroid hormones according to gestational age in pregnant Spanish women. BMC Res Notes. 2009;2:237. https://doi.org/10.1186/1756-0500-2-237.
72. Springer D, Zima T, Limanova Z. Reference intervals in evaluation of maternal thyroid function during the first trimester of pregnancy. Eur J Endocrinol. 2009;160:791–7. https://doi.org/10.1530/EJE-08-0890.
73. Männistö T, Surcel H-M, Ruokonen A, Vääräsmäki M, Pouta A, Bloigu A, Järvelin M-R, Hartikainen A-L, Suvanto E. Early pregnancy reference intervals of thyroid hormone concentrations in a thyroid antibody-negative pregnant population. Thyroid. 2011;21:291–8. https://doi.org/10.1089/thy.2010.0337.
74. Bliddal S, Feldt-Rasmussen U, Boas M, Faber J, Juul A, Larsen T, Precht DH. Gestational age-specific reference ranges from different laboratories misclassify pregnant women's thyroid status: comparison of two longitudinal prospective cohort studies. Eur J Endocrinol. 2014;170:329–39. https://doi.org/10.1530/EJE-13-0672.
75. Gao X, Li Y, Li J, Liu A, Sun W, Teng W, Shan Z. Gestational TSH and FT4 reference intervals in Chinese women: a systematic review and meta-analysis. Front Endocrinol (Lausanne). 2018;9:432. https://doi.org/10.3389/fendo.2018.00432.
76. Osinga JAJ, Derakhshan A, Feldt-Rasmussen U, Huang K, Vrijkotte TGM, Männistö T, Bassols J, López-Bermejo A, Aminorroaya A, Vafeiadi M, Broeren MAC, Palomaki GE, Ashoor G, Chen L, Lu X, Taylor PN, Tao FB, Brown SJ, Sitoris G, Chatzi L, Vaidya B, Popova PV, Vasukova EA, Kianpour M, Suvanto E, Grineva EN, Hattersley A, Pop VJM, Nelson SM, Walsh JP, Nicolaides KH, D'alton ME, Poppe KG, Chaker L, Bliddal S, Korevaar TIM. TSH and FT4 reference interval recommendations and prevalence of gestational thyroid dysfunction: quantification of current diagnostic approaches. J Clin Endocrinol Metab. 2024;109:868–78. https://doi.org/10.1210/clinem/dgad564.
77. Lafranchi SH. Thyroid function in preterm/low birth weight infants: impact on diagnosis and management of thyroid dysfunction. Front Endocrinol (Lausanne). 2021;12:666207. https://doi.org/10.3389/fendo.2021.666207.
78. Lafranchi S. Congenital hypothyroidism: etiologies, diagnosis, and management. Thyroid. 1999;9:735–40. https://doi.org/10.1089/thy.1999.9.735.
79. Ford G, Lafranchi SH. Screening for congenital hypothyroidism: a worldwide view of strategies. Best Pract Res Clin Endocrinol Metab. 2014;28:175–87. https://doi.org/10.1016/j.beem.2013.05.008.
80. Wassner AJ, Brown RS. Congenital hypothyroidism: recent advances. Curr Opin Endocrinol Diabetes Obes. 2015;22:407–12. https://doi.org/10.1097/MED.0000000000000181.

81. Wassner AJ. Congenital hypothyroidism. Clin Perinatol. 2018;45:1–18. https://doi.org/10.1016/j.clp.2017.10.004.
82. Darrat M, Kayes L, Woodside JV, Mullan K, Abid N. Congenital hypothyroidism in northern ireland: 40 years' experience of national screening programme. Clin Endocrinol. 2023;99:409–16. https://doi.org/10.1111/cen.14940.
83. Danner E, Jääskeläinen J, Niuro L, Huopio H, Niinikoski H, Viikari L, Kero J, Sund R. Comorbidity in congenital hypothyroidism—a nationwide, population-based cohort study. J Clin Endocrinol Metab. 2023;108:e1695–701. https://doi.org/10.1210/clinem/dgad334.
84. Grasberger H, Refetoff S. Resistance to thyrotropin. Best Pract Res Clin Endocrinol Metab. 2017;31:183–94. https://doi.org/10.1016/j.beem.2017.03.004.
85. Beck-Peccoz P, Rodari G, Giavoli C, Lania A. Central hypothyroidism—a neglected thyroid disorder. Nat Rev Endocrinol. 2017;13:588–98. https://doi.org/10.1038/nrendo.2017.47.
86. Donaldson MDC, Grosse SD. Does early identification of central congenital hypothyroidism result in improved outcomes. J Clin Endocrinol Metab. 2021;106:e2373–5. https://doi.org/10.1210/clinem/dgab059.
87. Lauffer P, Naafs JC, Bikker H, Garrelfs MR, Mooij CF, Boelen A, Zwaveling-Soonawala N, Van Trotsenburg ASP. Further delineation of central congenital hypothyroidism due to variants in tbl1x and irs4. Thyroid. 2023;33:880–4. https://doi.org/10.1089/thy.2022.0675.
88. Zhang HY, Wu FY, Zhang CX, Wu CY, Cui RJ, Liu XY, Yang L, Zhang Y, Sun F, Cheng F, Yang RM, Song HD, Zhao SX. Contactin 6, a novel causative gene for congenital hypothyroidism, mediates thyroid hormone biosynthesis through notch signaling. Thyroid. 2024;34:324–35. https://doi.org/10.1089/thy.2023.0594.
89. Monzani A, Prodam F, Rapa A, Moia S, Agarla V, Bellone S, Bona G. Endocrine disorders in childhood and adolescence: natural history of subclinical hypothyroidism in children and adolescents and potential effects of replacement therapy: a review. Eur J Endocrinol. 2013;168:R1–R11. https://doi.org/10.1530/EJE-12-0656.
90. Vigone MC, Capalbo D, Weber G, Salerno M. Mild hypothyroidism in childhood: who, when, and how should be treated. J Endocr Soc. 2018;2:1024–39. https://doi.org/10.1210/js.2017-00471.
91. Lazar L, Frumkin RB, Battat E, Lebenthal Y, Phillip M, Meyerovitch J. Natural history of thyroid function tests over 5 years in a large pediatric cohort. J Clin Endocrinol Metab. 2009;94:1678–82. https://doi.org/10.1210/jc.2008-2615.
92. Wasniewska M, Salerno M, Cassio A, Corrias A, Aversa T, Zirilli G, Capalbo D, Bal M, Mussa A, De Luca F. Prospective evaluation of the natural course of idiopathic subclinical hypothyroidism in childhood and adolescence. Eur J Endocrinol. 2009;160:417–21. https://doi.org/10.1530/EJE-08-0625.
93. Ittermann T, Thamm M, Wallaschofski H, Rettig R, Völzke H. Serum thyroid-stimulating hormone levels are associated with blood pressure in children and adolescents. J Clin Endocrinol Metab. 2012;97:828–34. https://doi.org/10.1210/jc.2011-2768.
94. Leung AKC, Leung AAC. Evaluation and management of the child with hypothyroidism. World J Pediatr. 2019;15:124–34. https://doi.org/10.1007/s12519-019-00230-w.
95. Walsh JP. Thyroid function across the lifespan: do age-related changes matter. Endocrinol Metab (Seoul). 2022;37:208–19. https://doi.org/10.3803/EnM.2022.1463.
96. De Andrade CLO, Alves C, Ramos HE. Congenital hypothyroidism and the deleterious effects on auditory function and language skills. Front Endocrinol (Lausanne). 2021;12:872.
97. Fernandez-Gonzalez SM, Perez Vila MM, Prado-Carro AM. Precocious puberty in hypothyroidism: mini-review of van wyk-grumbach syndrome. J Endocr Soc. 2023;7:bvad135. https://doi.org/10.1210/jendso/bvad135.
98. Kapelari K, Kirchlechner C, Hogler W, Schweitzer K, Virgolini I, Moncayo R. Pediatric reference intervals for thyroid hormone levels from birth to adulthood: a retrospective study. BMC Endocr Disord. 2008;8:15. https://doi.org/10.1186/1472-6823-8-15.

99. Iwaku K, Noh JY, Minagawa A, Kosuga Y, Suzuki M, Sekiya K, Matsumoto M, Ohye H, Kunii Y, Yoshihara A. Determination of pediatric reference levels of FT3, FT4 and TSH measured with eclusys kits. Endocr J. 2013;60:799–804.
100. Gammons S, Presley BK, White PC. Referrals for elevated thyroid stimulating hormone to pediatric endocrinologists. J Endocr Soc. 2019;3:2032–40. https://doi.org/10.1210/js.2019-00244.
101. Surup H, Vogel M, Koerner A, Hiemisch A, Oelkers L, Willenberg A, Kiess W, Kratzsch J. Pediatric reference intervals for thyrotropin, free triiodothyronine, and free thyroxine and the relevance of body mass index and puberty in measurement interpretation. Thyroid. 2021;31:1192–202. https://doi.org/10.1089/thy.2020.0780.
102. Lauffer P, Heinen CA, Goorsenberg AWM, Malekzadeh A, Henneman P, Heijboer AC, Zwaveling-Soonawala N, Boelen A, Van Trotsenburg ASP. Analysis of serum FT4 concentrations in healthy term neonates underlines need for local and laboratory-specific reference interval: a systematic review and meta-analysis of individual participant data. Thyroid. 2024; https://doi.org/10.1089/thy.2023.0562.
103. Mariotti S, Barbesino G, Caturegli P, Bartalena L, Sansoni P, Fagnoni F, Monti D, Fagiolo U, Franceschi C, Pinchera A. Complex alteration of thyroid function in healthy centenarians. J Clin Endocrinol Metab. 1993;77:1130–4.
104. Mariotti S, Franceschi C, Cossarizza A. The aging thyroid. Endocr Rev. 1995;16:686–715. https://doi.org/10.1210/edrv-16-6-686.
105. Monzani F, Del Guerra P, Caraccio N, Del Corso L, Casolaro A, Mariotti S, Pentimone F. Age-related modifications in the regulation of the hypothalamic-pituitary-thyroid axis. Horm Res. 1996;46:107–12.
106. Over R, Mannan S, Nsouli-Maktabi H, Burman KD, Jonklaas J. Age and the thyrotropin response to hypothyroxinemia. J Clin Endocrinol Metab. 2010;95:3675–83. https://doi.org/10.1210/jc.2010-0281.
107. Bowers J, Terrien J, Clerget-Froidevaux MS, Gothié JD, Rozing MP, Westendorp RGJ, Van Heemst D, Demeneix BA. Thyroid hormone signaling and homeostasis during aging. Endocr Rev. 2013;34:556–89. https://doi.org/10.1210/er.2012-1056.
108. Jansen SW, Roelfsema F, Van Der Spoel E, Akintola AA, Postmus I, Ballieux BE, Slagboom PE, Cobbaert CM, Van Der Grond J, Westendorp RG, Pijl H, Van Heemst D. Familial longevity is associated with higher TSH secretion and strong TSH-ft3 relationship. J Clin Endocrinol Metab. 2015;100:3806–13. https://doi.org/10.1210/jc.2015-2624.
109. Franceschi C, Ostan R, Mariotti S, Monti D, Vitale G. The aging thyroid: a reappraisal within the geroscience integrated perspective. Endocr Rev. 2019;40:1250–70. https://doi.org/10.1210/er.2018-00170.
110. Calsolaro V, Niccolai F, Pasqualetti G, Calabrese AM, Polini A, Okoye C, Magno S, Caraccio N, Monzani F. Overt and subclinical hypothyroidism in the elderly: when to treat. Front Endocrinol (Lausanne). 2019;10:177. https://doi.org/10.3389/fendo.2019.00177.
111. Tsai TY, Tu YK, Munir KM, Lin SM, Chang RH, Kao SL, Loh CH, Peng CC, Huang HK. Association of hypothyroidism and mortality in the elderly population: a systematic review and meta-analysis. J Clin Endocrinol Metab. 2020;105:1–13. https://doi.org/10.1210/clinem/dgz186.
112. Stott DJ, Rodondi N, Kearney PM, Ford I, Westendorp RGJ, Mooijaart SP, Sattar N, Aubert CE, Aujesky D, Bauer DC, Baumgartner C, Blum MR, Browne JP, Byrne S, Collet TH, Dekkers OM, Den Elzen WPJ, Du Puy RS, Ellis G, Feller M, Floriani C, Hendry K, Hurley C, Jukema JW, Kean S, Kelly M, Krebs D, Langhorne P, Mccarthy G, Mccarthy V, Mcconnachie A, Mcdade M, Messow M, O'flynn A, O'riordan D, Poortvliet RKE, Quinn TJ, Russell A, Sinnott C, Smit JWA, Van Dorland HA, Walsh KA, Walsh EK, Watt T, Wilson R, Gussekloo J, Trust SG. Thyroid hormone therapy for older adults with subclinical hypothyroidism. N Engl J Med. 2017;376:2534–44. https://doi.org/10.1056/NEJMoa1603825.

113. Holley M, Razvi S, Dew R, Maxwell I, Wilkes S. Assessing the cardiovascular effects of levothyroxine use in an ageing United Kingdom population (acel-uk) protocol: a cohort and target trial emulation study. Thyroid Res. 2023;16:43. https://doi.org/10.1186/s13044-023-00186-0.
114. Riis J, Westergaard L, Karmisholt J, Andersen SL, Andersen S. Biological variation in thyroid function tests in older adults and clinical implications. Clin Endocrinol. 2023;99:598–605. https://doi.org/10.1111/cen.14973.
115. Tan SY, Chubb SAP, Flicker L, Almeida OP, Golledge J, Hankey GJ, Yeap BB. Changes in thyroid function and evolution of subclinical thyroid disease in older men. Clin Endocrinol. 2024;100:170–80. https://doi.org/10.1111/cen.14997.
116. Bremner AP, Feddema P, Leedman PJ, Brown SJ, Beilby JP, Lim EM, Wilson SG, O'leary PC, Walsh JP. Age-related changes in thyroid function: a longitudinal study of a community-based cohort. J Clin Endocrinol Metab. 2012;97:1554–62. https://doi.org/10.1210/jc.2011-3020.
117. Vadiveloo T, Donnan PT, Murphy MJ, Leese GP. Age- and gender-specific TSH reference intervals in people with no obvious thyroid disease in tayside, scotland: the thyroid epidemiology, audit, and research study (tears). J Clin Endocrinol Metab. 2013;98:1147–53. https://doi.org/10.1210/jc.2012-3191.
118. Jonklaas J, Razvi S. Reference intervals in the diagnosis of thyroid dysfunction: treating patients not numbers. Lancet Diabetes Endocrinol. 2019;7:473–83. https://doi.org/10.1016/S2213-8587(18)30371-1.
119. Taylor PN, Lansdown A, Witczak J, Khan R, Rees A, Dayan CM, Okosieme O. Age-related variation in thyroid function—a narrative review highlighting important implications for research and clinical practice. Thyroid Res. 2023;16:7. https://doi.org/10.1186/s13044-023-00149-5.
120. Van Uytfanghe K, Ehrenkranz J, Halsall D, Hoff K, Loh TP, Spencer CA, Köhrle J. Thyroid stimulating hormone and thyroid hormones (triiodothyronine and thyroxine): an American Thyroid Association-commissioned review of current clinical and laboratory status. Thyroid. 2023;33:1013–28. https://doi.org/10.1089/thy.2023.0169.

GPSR Compliance

The European Union's (EU) General Product Safety Regulation (GPSR) is a set of rules that requires consumer products to be safe and our obligations to ensure this.

If you have any concerns about our products, you can contact us on ProductSafety@springernature.com

In case Publisher is established outside the EU, the EU authorized representative is:

Springer Nature Customer Service Center GmbH
Europaplatz 3
69115 Heidelberg, Germany

Batch number: 10732090

Printed by Printforce, the Netherlands